PURE SMART LIFE

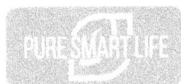

RESET YOUR LIFE
FOR A HEALTHY YOU

Understanding Guide in Taking the 1st Steps on a healing
wellness plan for a Healthier Lifestyle: Includes Meal Plan,
Healing the Inside, Fitness, Mindset, & much more...

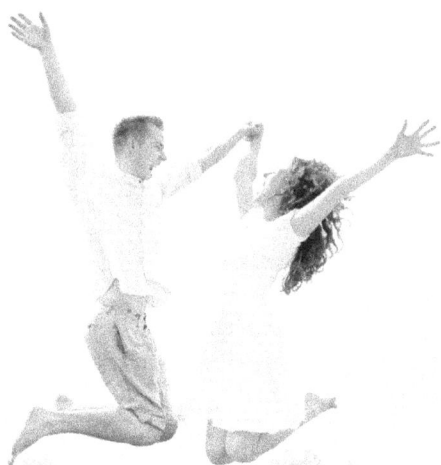

Pure Smart Life

RESET YOUR LIFE FOR A HEALTHY YOU

UNDERSTANDING GUIDE IN TAKING THE 1ST STEPS ON A HEALING WELLNESS PLAN FOR A HEALTHIER LIFESTYLE: INCLUDES MEAL PLAN, HEALING THE INSIDE, FITNESS, MINDSET, & MUCH MORE…

PURE SMART LIFE

Amazing
3AQ Products, LLC

DEDICATION

For my Family

CONTENTS

BOOK DESCRIPTION

Learn how to take your health, youth, and happiness back into your hands with techniques that target the very source of every problem under the sun!

Do you feel like you're swimming under an ocean of unexplained health issues, or are you the "lucky one" who has a list of prescription medicine as long as the letters in the ingredients you can't pronounce?

Are you tired of being exhausted? Are you sick of being unwell? The cycle never ends, and your life isn't what its potential could be. Being unwell is one thing, but having doctors poke and prod you like cattle is another.

Your medicine cabinet fills up, and yet, you feel no better. Your chronic conditions are climbing in volume and intensity, but no one can tell you why! Sometimes, it's a nagging feeling we get in the pit of our stomachs that says: "Hey, something's wrong!"

Yet, the endless swarm of medical experts are stumped. You know your body, and you know when something isn't right anymore. Your brain is smart enough to know that your current lifestyle isn't the one you want.

Being tired, bloated, overweight, frequently down with the flu, and having doctors pile more medicine that isn't working for you is no better than trying to grow a tree without planting the seed first.

How long does your body take to recover from every setback? How much of your life is disrupted by prolonged recoveries and frequent illnesses? **What if I told you that you could stop everything from worsening?**

You wouldn't believe how easy it is to combat some of the most common chronic ailments. **You have no idea of the self-healing power your body and mind possess.** Best of all, you can turn back the clock to sustain your age, vibrancy, and happiness.

Whoever said there was no fountain of youth, clearly didn't know the secrets inside the body, the same secrets that science reveals daily, but we're too blind to see them. Taking back control of your health is as simple as learning about these practical secrets.

After a few tweaks, some practical exercises, and simple lifestyle changes, you'll be among the top contenders for optimal health. Your entire family is going to thank you, just as mine did. This journey is one for everyone—kids, older people, and young adults.

This lifestyle jumpstart will include:

- **Every secret** the food and medical industries fail to share
- The effects of daily products on our health
- The evolution of food and how it sets our bodies off track

- The **source of every disease** you can imagine
- **Six** tests that look for the **real roots** of your problems
- Alternative cleanses to remove harmful substances from your body
- Cleaning your system abruptly or for the long haul
- **22 nutritional tricks** to boost your health and diminish symptoms
- **14 natural hacks** you can buy anywhere
- What the **real superfoods** are
- **12 personal favorite recipes** that can't be found elsewhere
- A meal-plan as simple as they come
- A professional guide to **tricking your body into burning its own fat**
- **19 workouts** that reset your body and health
- The art of applying the mind, body, and soul connection

It's time for your body to reset itself to the natural self-healing, self-promoting, and disease-killing mode it once was. Natural doesn't mean you need to forget science or ancient beliefs; instead, you'll use these valuable tools to kickstart your system again. *The time is now!* Click on the purchase button, and let's get started!

COPYRIGHT

Just for you !

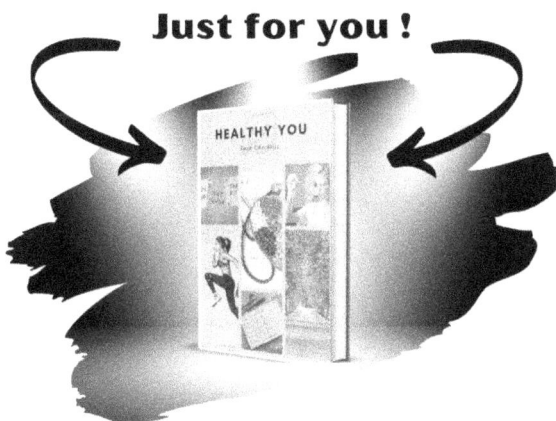

A Special Gift to our Readers

Included with your purchases out Task Checklist Guide to help you on your journey. This step-by-step task guide will prepare you in getting the correct steps in getting healthy.

Click the link below and let us know which email address to send it too.

Healthy You - Task Checklist

www.amazingjaqproducts.com/publishing/HealthyYou

INTRODUCTION

Henry Ward Beecher once said: "The body is like a piano, and happiness is like music. It's needful to have the instrument in good order."

I'm sure you've had days where you wake up and your music sounds like a clowder of cats meowing, each to their own tune. You take a step toward your medicine cabinet with the bottles popping out of it. This doesn't mean that you're old either. Young and old alike are suffering from chronic disorders daily. Pain, inflammation, fatigue, light-headedness, digestive issues, and more serious conditions are only a diagnosis away.

Unfortunately, they're not always diagnosed either. Some people consider themselves lucky when their doctors have listed a myriad of disorders, ranging from high blood pressure to depression. They feel temporarily relieved as they pop those pills like candy. It's becoming more and more common for younger crowds to suffer from diabetes, insulin resistance, and severe conditions inflicting their hearts and other major organs.

Western medicine swamps us with treatments, tests, and follow-ups. However, what do you tell the doctor when his treatments have made no difference in your life? You still feel like a dog in the gutter. You still experience pain, and the worst of all is that your doctor can't tell you why you're in pain. At some point, you must consider the fact that maybe, just maybe, your doctor doesn't have the natural knowledge to help you.

Instead, he sends you for another list of tests that come back with nothing! Your legs keep swelling, you can't lose weight, and your digestive problems are brushed off as some form of irritable bowel syndrome (IBS). Your life is miserable because your music doesn't change, even after the doctor tunes your piano over and over. The treatments keep coming, and suddenly, you have another disorder.

All you wanted, originally, was to decrease the bloating in your stomach or lose a few pounds. You wanted a chance at leading a healthier lifestyle. Heck, you've probably tried a few methods already. Yes, that includes chewing on celery to burn more calories than you're eating. You've been to a nutritionist, but they were probably the wrong one. Finally, we have the people who feel well but have a nagging sensation that bothers them.

Maybe you can't call yourself sick, but you're tired of suffering from the common cold 10 times a year. Your sinuses act up, and your allergies are the worst! Our health doesn't start with chronic conditions. It also doesn't begin with severe symptoms. It starts with a strange sensation after eating. It starts when you run after a cab and realize that you're breathless. Heck, you're 28 and breathless in the middle of New York City.

Our health changes after we gain a few pounds and

someone mentions it. Standing in front of the mirror, squeezing the roll that seemed to form overnight, we wonder where the hell we went wrong. Many people think they lead healthy lifestyles. They follow the fad diets and push their bodies to the ultimate exercise limits. Half the time, they're doing it all wrong because they don't understand the foundation of healthy living.

Life is formidable, and your health is as fragile as the human ego. The human body is capable of great things, but it can also work against us when we don't look after it. If only you knew how simple it was to maintain the best health and prevent chronic disorders. If only you knew how easy it was to take back control and tune your piano perfectly. Everything starts in the same place—inside the body and mind.

Your body has the ability to rejuvenate itself, maintain youth, and flush the unwanted products into the toilet where they belong. Do you suffer from life-changing chronic illnesses like cancer, heart disease, or kidney failure? I'll never say that a cancer patient must stop their chemotherapy, but they can use their body's natural fight against it to lessen the symptoms and give themselves a better chance of overcoming it.

They can learn what to avoid and what to consume. Well, restoring the body to its natural state is how you dissipate the symptoms of these conditions. Resetting the body can even prevent serious or minor health concerns in the future, for the young and old. Your body already has everything it needs, but years of unknown abuse is what's prevented it from sustaining a perfect balance. The same applies to any disorder.

There's a sad truth in the world. Did you know that there are 10,000 diseases listed globally, but there are only 500 cures (Kessler, 2016)? That's shocking, to say the least. Western medicine and modern nutrition have failed you. That's why 133 million or 40% of the American population had multiple chronic disorders in 2014 (National Health Council, 2014). These disorders ranged from IBS to depression to heart disease. It included every one of the 10,000 diseases known.

Obesity is also a chronic disorder unless you lose weight. The proof is always in the pudding, though. More than one-third of Americans are now relying on natural or alternative lifestyles, including medicine, nutrition, and treatments (Wong, 2004). America is very sick right now, but there are so many natural methods of returning your body to its original state.

You were born with the innate ability to fight disease, consume natural foods, and live until a ripe age. It starts with removing the chemicals, foods, and toxins you've been exposed to. There are so many modern food products and medicine tainted with chemicals that our ancestors would've flushed down the drain. The products are found in nearly everything, and I'll show you where to look.

Certain products work against the body's natural immunity. They tear down your defenses and leave you susceptible to health problems. You'll be surprised where these ingredients are found because it isn't only in your food. I'm going to share some scientific knowledge with you about the body and its systems, from the head to the toes. Everything plays a role inside of you, and you're in for trouble if you're not looking after it.

There are some mystery ailments triggered by simple biological responses and other illnesses that aren't even recognized in western medicine. You're going to learn how toxic your body has become and how to test for precise culprits so that you can design a personal journey back to health. Various detoxes can help you remove these toxins before you apply your new lifestyle.

I'm going to teach you what clean eating really means because too many people are confused about it. There are dos and don'ts you need to know about, or the body's response to your new food choices won't make a difference. I've shared my secret recipes with you so that you can take inspiration from them, and I've given you an idea for a weekly food planner.

You'll find natural remedies so that you can stop pumping your blood full of unnecessary medications. Fasting is discussed comprehensively so that you can cater it to your life. Healthy living is far from boring. It's filled with excitement, experimentation, and funny mistakes. The mistakes are harmless, anyway. You'll also learn about a myriad of exercises that help your body jump start again.

Some exercises are simple, others push your boundaries, but they are all affordable and space-saving. You'll skip nothing as you apply the final tricks to repair the mind so that it can't alter the body anymore. Your journey will take you to better health, improved happiness, and a life worth living. I've been where you are now in so many ways. I was even adamant that I was leading a healthy life as it was.

I thought I ate right, remained active, and led my family down a path of wholesome living, but I still suffered from simple irritants that grew into larger health problems. My kids were always getting sick at certain times of the year, missing school, and keeping my wife and me on our toes. It was either allergies, colds, influenza, stomach bugs, or anything making the rounds.

However, my idea of healthy living was finally shattered when my daughter was diagnosed with chronic inflammatory demyelinating polyneuropathy (CIPD), making her life anything but pleasant. It's a condition where the myelin surrounding the nerve fibers are worn down. Imagine nerve pain, imagine inflammation around the nerves from an injury, and now, imagine my little girl with this condition.

I needed answers yesterday, and so I set out on a 10-year journey, studying the true source of healthy living. My goal is for my entire family, including my little girl and me, to be healthy, fit, disease-free, and symptom-free. It didn't take long before the smallest of changes were shining through the family. I finally realized that the kids went two years without getting sick or missing school.

It doesn't take a truck of changes to see a difference, but the more you add, the more you benefit. My passion for answers led me to medical, holistic, and biological pathways. I'm determined to be healthy and to see that my family remains so, too. I'm also determined to help you realize what's going on. Being unwell and not living the life you deserve isn't normal.

I share my experience, knowledge, and passion with you so that you can do with it what you need to. Are you ready to change your health status? Are you determined to overcome chronic symptoms? Are you willing to live healthily in the true definition of it? Then, I suggest you keep reading to learn about the practical changes you can implement forthwith.

OH, IT'S JUST A VIRUS!

Chapter 1

You have this idea that you're eating right, following a healthy lifestyle, and watching your calories to try your best to keep your weight down and heart-healthy. Most people brush their colds off because it's just a common virus. The fact that they're stuck in bed for a week, multiple times a year, taking more time from work than their sick days allow, and missing out on the exciting parts of life every time they fall ill is certainly not just a virus.

You can't believe what's happening in your body while you think you're eating healthy and avoiding viruses with every means you have. If only you knew what was really going on when you felt unwell. You can continue thinking that your lifestyle is profoundly balanced, or you can dig deeper to unveil the mysteries of disease and its connection to food.

The Lying Food Industry

Everyone knows the foundation of healthy eating, right? Whole foods, healthy fats, fruits, and vegetables are echoed whenever we think of eating right. Slap a salad together, throw some strawberries on top, and call me healthy. But wait, are these products perfectly safe, or do you need to know more? One of the biggest lies you've ever been told is that fruit and vegetables are safe, healthy, and life-promoting. It's more complicated than simply wrapping your commercially-raised chicken breast in lettuce and spreading some tomatoes around the edges.

You need to start thinking about food in a different light, even the so-called healthy options. Food was so much simpler a few decades back. There were no chemical processes, pesticides, and harmful substances added to our food to speed up the harvesting process and keep pests at bay. Okay, the world's population has exploded, but is that an excuse to poison our food? The centers for disease control (CDC) have released frightening figures that make us wonder whether our food is getting healthier or whether it's taking away from us.

Autism is impacting one in every 50 children, 74% of Americans are overweight, 36% of them obese, and there's been a 71% increase in Alzheimer's disease since 2000 (Living Young, 2019). Do these figures make sense when you learn that Monsanto's Roundup Herbicide was sprayed enough in 2014 to cover every acre of ground with eight pounds of pesticide? That's only the agricultural number because the same pesticide is used on lawns, school grounds, and public parks. Monsanto claims that their pesticide contains no human-activated chemicals.

This is nothing but a big, fat lie! They argue that the mechanisms used to kill pests are absent in humans. The mechanism is called the shikimate pathway, which is used by bacteria, fungi, and parasites to move through the plant's biological

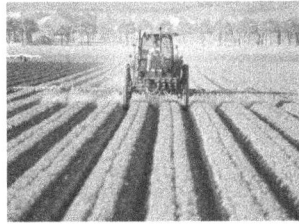

Pesticides

structure. Humans also have bacteria in their gut that needs to move through an inevitable shikimate pathway that extends along the entire endocrine system. The endocrine system even connects to the central nervous system (CNS) in the brain and along the spine, and is responsible for our metabolism. The gut and brain are connected like opposite ends of a magnet.

Monsanto didn't account for the millions of bacteria evident in the human gut. In fact, there are multiple bits of bacteria living in the stomach for every cell in the body. Understanding the balance that we require in our gut bacteria can be seen when doctors prescribe probiotics to counter the effects of antibiotics. The bacteria's role in your stomach is critical to your immune system and everything attached to it. Nevertheless, glyphosate is the main ingredient in Roundup and it's known as a carcinogen. A carcinogen triggers body cell deformity to cause abnormal structures, and it's often seen in cancer patients. The pesticide residue in our agricultural produce is monitored, but glyphosate isn't.

Glyphosate is the first of many enemies. It harms the body by attracting more food-borne toxins and chemicals once your cells start shifting into abnormalities. It upsets the stomach bacteria which is responsible for many good processes in the body. Even worse, it targets the good bacteria only. Now, the bad bacteria called pathogens can flourish and induce diseases. Chronic inflammation starts, and the good bacteria aren't there to counter the harmful effects of it. Inflammation is good under normal circumstances, but long-term inflammation is more harmful than you can believe.

Suddenly, the climate within your body is set for diseases, such as autism in children, allergies, cancer, cardiovascular disease, infertility, and obesity. It can also cause Alzheimer's, depression, multiple sclerosis (MS), amyotrophic lateral sclerosis (ALS), inflammatory bowel disease (IBD), Crohn's disease, and colitis. The fallout isn't limited to these chronic conditions either because abnormal cells in the body can lead to just about any condition as the immune system is confused. So, do you still think that fruit and vegetables are healthy options?

Well, they can be if you're eating organic produce or growing your own. Even barley, grains, and wheat need to be organic. Keep in mind that some organic products are also sprayed with "organic pesticides." Be careful of what you buy, and make sure it hasn't been poisoned with glyphosate or other hidden chemicals. Pesticides aren't the only enemy. Our food has taken many blows to its health definition in the race to produce more food, faster, and preserve it for longer. Processed food is easily available, tastes great with all the harmful enhancements made to it, and is sadly addictive. It's no lie that processed food tastes better, but that's why you're hooked on it.

The happiness part of your brain is flooded with dopamine to make you want more. Some food additives and processed junk are as addictive as heroin. Refined sugar is just one of the culprits. Unfortunately, processed food is pumped full of sugar, salt, preservatives, dangerous fats, and chemicals to make agricultural processing faster. For example, non-organic farmers hasten the harvest by chemically inducing the drying process of grains. Instead of waiting for the grains to dry naturally, they spray them to speed up the process. Mechanical processing will always be part of our agriculture, but chemical processing is dangerous.

Whole foods have a simple method of identification. Their labels contain a single ingredient. Look at the label on the strawberries before you buy it. Does it only say strawberries or is there a list of additives, preservatives, and ingredients you can't even pronounce? The longer the ingredient list stretches, the more the product has been chemically processed. Some processing is even hidden in plain sight. Almonds are known to be healthy and offer many great benefits, but only until they've been processed and refined to an unrecognizable point.

Look at the ingredients label again, and try to convince yourself that almonds are still healthy when the word is followed by vegetable oil, sugar, and salt. Raw almonds are healthy, but chocolate-coated, wasabi, lime-chili, and sriracha almonds are bad news. There are too many harmful additives and ingredients to eat food that lists ingredients as long as Route 66. Processed food contains mountains of sugar. Another sugar you must be aware of is called high-fructose corn syrup, which is also found in processed foods. Sugar is an empty calorie that only builds fat in the liver and abdomen. It gives you no nutrients, and it destabilizes your insulin levels, cholesterol, and metabolism.

Artificial additives are used to make food last longer, more colorfully attractive, and to taste better. The scariest part of additives is that food companies don't need to divulge ingredients because it's their secret recipe. They don't have to tell you what you're eating. Aspartame is one artificial sweetener that's been in the limelight for weight gain and hormonal imbalances in the body, and it's found in many sugar-free sodas and "health products." The body needs carbohydrates, but the type of carb we eat is what matters. Unfortunately, processed food contains refined carbs that are easily digested as simple carbs, leaving you craving more. Carbohydrates also play a role in energy and glucose/insulin levels. You should stick to complex carbs found in whole foods.

Chemical processing also kills the nutrients and vitamins your body needs. The food industry combats this by adding synthetic alternatives, but the replacement falls short of the body's requirements. The more you eat processed foods, the less you're benefiting from the natural nutrients, vitamins, and antioxidants your body needs to sustain health. Fiber is also diminished in processed food, and it's not only bad for your bowel movements. Fiber is food for the good bacteria in the stomach. A lack of fiber leads to obesity because you're not sufficed long enough if you don't eat organic fiber. That's why bread only keeps you satisfied for a short period.

Finally, processed food contains enormous amounts of unhealthy fats from corn, sunflower, canola, and vegetable oils. The reason why these fats are unhealthy is that they're hydrogenated. This means that they've been turned from a liquid into a semi-solid state to prolong shelf-life. Now, the fat turns into a trans fat, which raises your triglycerides to promote bad cholesterol. Trans fat also contains omega-6, which causes oxidation and inflammation in the body. It can lead to heart disease, and consuming excessive amounts of processed food is like scooping margarine from the tub into your mouth. Trans fats aren't found in butter, olive oil, and coconut oil, though.

Everything you consume impacts your body, immune system, metabolic system, and the ability to lead a long, happy life. The food industry tries to solve population and demand problems, but the effects aren't justified. Everything starts with good intentions but unfolds into harmful consequences. Processed foods and pesticides are only the tips of the iceberg, but they can cause unhealthy problems that shorten our lives.

Mysterious Ailments

The relationship between your stomach and the rest of your body, including your brain, is undeniably responsible for the times you get the flu thrice throughout winter. Your body is trying to defend itself, but this unravels in illnesses and irritations. What about all the illnesses that can't be cured? Why are there so many misunderstood diseases when doctors can fill a prescription for just about anything? Instead, you suffer from symptoms, some of which are easily recognized and others that are pushed aside as having a down day.

Light-headedness, fatigue, cognitive problems, and headaches are simply part of life some days, right? Depression, anxiety, tremors, body aches, palpitations, tingles, and numbness come and go, and nobody knows any better. Well, health-conscious people know that these symptoms are stirred by underlying problems, many of which start in the stomach. Have you ever wondered why pain exists? There are two kinds, namely acute and chronic. Acute pain is the sudden jolt of unpleasant sensations in your body when you kick your toe against the table.

An immediate response is triggered in the immune system that extends through billions of tiny nerve endings. Nerve endings warn us about anything harmful or dangerous, and they connect to the brain to start what's called the fight or fix response. The brain then sends signals to various glands and organs to produce the immune response that causes inflammation and the repair of the damaged tissue. So, pain and inflammation are the body's way of showing that it's fixing the problem. Pain is a good sign because it prevents further damage. However, pain becomes a problem when it's chronic and exists for a long time.

This means that the immune response hasn't stopped working. It's easy to feel overwhelmed when you have pain, but there's no indication of damage to body tissue. Chronic pain isn't a response to immediate danger. It happens when the body's immune system has flipped the switch to repair mode, but there's nothing to repair. The immune system can also be tricked by abnormal cells that look damaged, making it work overtime. This is how chronic inflammation starts gathering too. The immune system and brain will always try to fix, fight, or erase foreign-looking cells, even if it sends the body into self-destruct mode.

Pain can be as subtle as having a stomach cramp after eating too much, or it can be as dire as a siren ringing constantly. How can you stop the pain or the inflammatory response from happening? You can't always cover the screeching siren with aspirin because this only ignores the problem. Acute pain is treatable with aspirin, but the chronic reaction in your body needs to be treated differently or the immune response will continue whether you like it or not. The cause of the problem needs to be addressed. What's causing abnormalities in your cells, and what's triggering the prolonged immune response? Some disorders are so mysterious that doctors and scientists can't easily detect the reason for your chronic response.

Without detection, how can you treat it? Why not use the body's natural healing ability to counter the reaction instead? Irrespective, you'd still have to use specialty tests to determine what's causing the immune system to stay in the fight or fix reaction. You'll learn about the specialty tests soon. However, the evidence that modern medicine can't treat or even detect the cause of many disorders that remain a mystery is the reason why we need to holistically allow the body to heal itself and maintain its own health. We can influence it from the outside with the foods we eat and the lifestyles we lead, but adding a flux of modern medicine isn't always the answer. Even doctors confirm that some conditions can't be treated.

They can slow some down, and they can minimize the symptoms, but they can't stop the immune system's response in every case. Only you can do this by teaching your body to relax the response and use it only for real threats. Some mysterious diseases still plague modern medicine, becoming more and more common among unhealthy people who think that they're leading healthy lifestyles.

Acquired Immune Deficiency Syndrome (AIDS) isn't an African continent problem. It exists everywhere, and you can't even tell who has it anymore because modern medicine suppressed the fallout symptoms now. There's still no cure, and it remains a potent killer worldwide, especially in developing countries.

Alzheimer's disease is a degenerative brain disorder and not just forgetfulness. It's vastly misunderstood, but the body's immune response that attacks cells wrongly perceived as threats can be a reason why numbers have escalated over the last few decades.

The common cold might be the most annoying illness we can suffer from, but it still can't be treated or cured with medicine.

Avian Flu is one of the deadliest viruses, but we can't cure it. The body starts the immune response that causes inflammation, and the best chance we have is to focus on the reaction in our bodies.

The Pica virus makes people crave substances they can't consume because their bodies need nutrients and vitamins that aren't in the stomach. The brain is starved by the gut and sends signals to make you crave dirt, paper, clay, and even glue.

Autoimmune disorders like MS and Lupus don't need much explanation. The name says it all because the immune system attacks healthy cells that it wrongly sees as threats. Eventually, the immune system turns on healthy organs because it sees them as alien invaders. Autoimmune diseases can't be cured with medicine; doctors can only treat the symptoms.

Schizophrenia must be the most misunderstood mental disorder out there. People struggle to distinguish between reality and fantasy while suffering from delusions, hallucinations, and mood instability. It also can't be cured and is only treated for symptoms.

Creutzfeldt-Jakob Disease, or better known as mad cow disease, is another rare and untreatable brain disorder. Doctors can't prevent the casualties from it, and they can't pinpoint the exact location either. It also starts as an immune response throughout the body and mind.

Chronic fatigue syndrome is another medical mystery. It can be so intense that you're stuck in bed for days, but there's no way of traditionally testing for it unless you rule out every other possible cause of the immune response.

Morgellons Disease is something from nightmares as people feel a crawling or tingling sensation under their skin. The sensations are caused by nerve endings, being rather similar to the immune response too.

These diseases gobsmack scientists, but they all contain a hint of commonality. The body goes into the fight or fixed response. Whatever causes the immune response is often unknown, but the brain and body fight to repair healthy organs and cells, leading to the opposite effect. The longer the body attacks healthy cells, the more likely they are to become unhealthy.

We have a new disease in our midst as well, and it's targeting our children. Coronavirus-disease 2019 or COVID-19 has certainly thrown the world upside down. At first, children were thought to have the greatest immunity toward it, but it wasn't long before children started ending up in critical care, and I say this with a knob in my throat, but some have passed away. It started in the United Kingdom (UK) when 12 young children became critical, and followed in New York when another three kids were lost to the dreaded immune response that was seemingly triggered by COVID-19 (O'Neill, 2020).

COVID-19 is vastly misunderstood, but it's proven to attack the immune system, causing the fight or fix response to work overtime, and in some cases, lead to the penultimately unwanted result. It seems to attack children under five more, and this might be due to their immune systems being fragile and underdeveloped. The New York children aged five, seven, and 18 experienced a response in their bodies that was similar to an old and rare condition called Kawasaki Disease. It started with a fever and rash before it led to inflammation of the blood vessels and tissue surrounding major organs. The link between COVID-19 and the autoimmune response is still being studied as the virus continues to evade cure.

The new disorder has been called the pediatric-multi system inflammatory syndrome. The direct connection to COVID-19 remains speculative, but if it's anything like Kawasaki Disease, children will be at risk for heart disease and brain aneurysms when they grow older thanks to the inflammation that damaged their blood vessels. This new condition has even shown similarities to known autoimmune diseases because the constant flux of inflammation damages organs throughout the body, or at the very least, it withers and ages them. Before confirming the possibility of the condition being connected to COVID-19, it was established that all the presenting patients either tested positive or had antibodies, meaning that they already recovered from COVID-19.

There's too much mystery in the medical world. Moreover, the food industry is always trying to justify their reasons for processing our food and spraying it full of pesticides. It isn't justified when you remember the gut-brain connection. Improving your health mentally, physically, and emotionally has much to do with this brain-gut connection, and it can be used to eat healthily and keep your immune system tame.

MORE TOXINS! WHAT'S REALLY HAPPENING IN YOUR BODY?

Chapter 2

Toxins are everywhere! It's no wonder we feel stressed when we learn about the body, gut, brain, and healthy lifestyles. It doesn't help us to stay under a rock and keep eating what we do, though. Learning about toxicity and what it does to the body only broadens your awareness so that you can implement changes in your lifestyle and think about food in new ways. Ignoring the problem has never worked for anyone, so push through a little longer. It's time you learned about what's going on inside your body.

The Vast Microbiome

How small and insignificant I feel when I stare at the night sky that stretches further than my eyes can see. The stars can't be counted in this infinite universe and neither can the synaptic connections in your brain. Most people have a good understanding of the complexity and infinite reach of the connections in our brains, and they know that counting the stars is as fruitful as counting the grains of sand on a beach. Now, what many people don't know is that the gut is just as vast as the night sky. There's a network called the microbiome that extends throughout your small and large intestines. It's made up of trillions of bacteria that outnumber the body's cells by 100 to one (Cresci & Izzo, 2019).

The entire gastrointestinal tract is laden with bacteria that play a major role in your body, and this collection is called the microbiome. This network is connected to every part of your body, regulating many functions, and keeping your hormones and electrolytes in check. The research in Cresci and Izzo's paper confirms that every aspect has been studied because systems this complex need to be understood. The imbalance of the good bacteria or microbiome has been connected to IBS, IBD, obesity, type two diabetes, and atopy. Atopy is when our bodies become sensitive to certain stimulants, and we develop an allergy. Atopy also happens when we suffer from asthma and eczema.

The kidneys aren't exempt from the disaster that befalls us when we consume excessive toxins that set the microbiome off balance. The kidneys play an important role in ridding our bodies of toxins, but they can't

Gut Bacteria

do this without the help of the friendly bacteria in the digestive tract. The bacteria help by breaking down the composition of the food we eat and pushes toxins into the kidneys where water flushes it out. The liver plays a similar role where the toxins are collected after bacterial reconstruction has separated the toxins from the nutritious parts of your

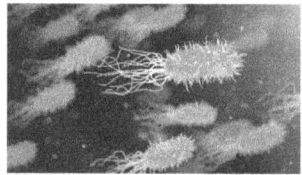

food. The liver is a key player in detoxification and moving toxins out of the body.

The toxins will be pushed through the skin to clear more space when the liver can't handle the influx anymore. This leads to acne, eczema, and even jaundice. Jaundice is a yellow-tinted skin that indicates serious problems in the liver. The liver and kidneys can only handle so many toxins, and if we aren't keeping the bacteria healthy, then we might as well quit on these two major organs. Water flushes the kidneys and keeps the gut bacteria's job to a minimum. Harmful gut bacteria floods the kidneys with uremic toxins that accumulate and impact the immune system when they can't process them anymore.

Gut bacteria also have functions that encourage the balance of the brain-immune system connection. They collect the nutrients the brain and other organs need. Bacteria also synthesize amino acids and enzymes. Amino acids are crucial to the oxygen levels traveling through your bloodstream, and enzymes are proteins that assist the metabolism in changing cells into energy to keep your body and immune system functioning at its peak. The metabolism is also responsible for your weight. The microbiome can keep diseases at bay, and it helps the body to fight real threats when the immune system attacks genuine problems. So, having bad bacteria overpower the good guys doesn't only cause inflammation and pain.

It can set off a cycle within your body that even affects the mind. Bacteria exist on your skin, in your mouth, and placenta, but the majority of it resides in the gut. Not every reaction to poor bacterial maintenance is as extreme as inflammation that restricts your arteries and pushes your cholesterol up. You'll physically look as poor as your insides have become if toxic levels get too high. Your metabolism slows down because it's so overworked already that the intended glands in your body can't regulate your digestion anymore. Now, you can add some additional weight to the acne to make yourself fit the insides you've encouraged.

I don't mean this as an insult to anyone, but no one wants to be obese with acne that covers their face and back to map the lifestyle they lead. The brain is a primary point of interest because it's responsible for regulating hormones and chemicals in your body that are required for critical functions. The adrenal glands are instructed by the pineal gland in the brain to release cortisol and adrenaline. These hormones are often called the enemy of people, but they also have a job. Nothing in the body is there to harm us, it's us that harms the body with toxic food and products. The CNS under attack is where Alzheimer's and Parkinson's Disease incubate in the brain.

Keeping your toxin levels too high is like playing target practice with your brain cells and hitting each one that you aim for. The relationship between the gut and brain is so complicated, fragile, and intricate that researchers keep looking for answers. Medical experts know that the stomach, intestines, and colon can be the cause of diseases, and they've established that it's our intake that offsets the balance in this fragile system (Ghaisais et al., 2016). Medication, stress, activity levels, and food are all to blame for hitting the microbiome with a baseball bat.

Researchers agree on one thing; the only way to restore the balance and stop the body from attacking its own organs is to balance the microbiome with whole foods, natural products, and lifestyle changes that encourage the bacteria to flourish healthily.

Signs of Toxicity

Toxicity presents itself in many horrible ways. I started with signs that were easy to dismiss as the ebb and flow of life because who suspects unexplained mild headaches as a sign? At 45, my symptoms started snowballing into depression, cognitive restraints, and body aches that made no sense. Numbness and tingling also prevailed slowly, and I began questioning my health. The symptoms weren't present all of the time and were mild enough to be irritations sometimes. Nonetheless, I needed to know why my body was feeling dreadful at such a young age when I led a relatively healthy lifestyle.

My entire family led a healthy lifestyle in our minds, but it wasn't until my daughter's inflammatory problems that I noticed symptoms that didn't make sense, so I began my research. Unfortunately, most general practitioners don't understand body toxicity in-depth unless it's mentioned or an investigation is requested. However, some signs poke their heads out when we feel off and don't know why.

You Can't Shake the Weight

Don't echo the old saying that you're big boned or genetically predisposed to being overweight. Ask yourself whether you've been leading a healthy, nutritious lifestyle, counting calories, and watching your weight, but you still can't shake the love handles or flatten your stomach. You could have an excess of lipophilic toxins stored in your fatty cells as they can't survive in normal cells. These toxins preserve themselves to survive, and that's why you can't lose weight. They include polychlorinated biphenyl (PCB), which is a chemical residue from pesticides. Chemical dioxins are even more toxic because they impact the brain and reproductive systems. These pesticidal toxins can make it seem impossible to lose weight.

You're Always Tired

How often do you sleep for eight hours at night and still wake up feeling exhausted? It's not in your head because it could also be due to toxins. Toxicity can increase your stress levels, making your adrenal glands release too much adrenaline. Your body is then always working overtime, and you reach adrenal fatigue. Coffee stimulates adrenaline as well, so think of it as drinking far too much coffee and becoming wired. Your heart rate increases and palpitations lead to short bursts of blood being pumped throughout your body. There isn't enough time to recycle oxygen into carbon-dioxide and expel it from the body either. That's why you become tired, breathless, and experience fast heartbeats when you exert yourself just a little bit. Getting out of bed with adrenal fatigue is already exhausting.

You Can't Sleep

The release of the cortisol and adrenaline hormones can also cause the opposite effect when your body and mind are in constant alertness. You struggle to sleep and suffer from insomnia. Cortisol is supposed to be running at higher levels in the morning so that you can start your day. It's the stress hormone, but it also makes you awake and alert. It's supposed to be lowest in the evenings, but can be high with a toxic imbalance of hormones in your body. Insomnia also worsens your health, making this a double-sided blade.

Your Thoughts Are Fuzzy

Fuzzy thoughts are blamed on toxicity, too, when your monosodium glutamate (MSG) and aspartame flavor enhancers are at new highs. Unfortunately, MSG is stuffed into most food products even though it's naturally present in low doses in some fruits and vegetables. It's the processed amounts that hit you hard. MSG is an excitotoxin that acts as a natural amino acid to promote the health of your neuro-transmitters in the brain. Neurotransmitters are the connec-tions between one neuron and another that sends instructions along the line to glands within the brain and body. Too much MSG, which means anything more than the natural amounts you must consume, is a recipe for foggy thoughts because the neurotransmitters break down after overworking them. Aspartame and MSG excite your brainy cells into submission, and they can die.

You Have Unexplained Headaches

Aspartame and MSG are to blame for this one too. The excitement happening in your brain is exhausting for the connections, and this leads to headaches. Other chemicals that cause unexplained migraines are heavy metals, preserv-atives, and artificial coloring.

Your Moods Swing Like a Bat

Mood swings are a sure sign that your hormones are out of sync, as any doctor will tell you. Xenoestrogens are one chemical byproduct found in pesticides, plastic, and chem-ical processing that imitates estrogen in the body. Estrogen is an important compound in the body that regulates moods, menstrual cycles, and even hair growth. It also acts as part of the reproductive cycle in men and women. Its influence on your emotional well-being is stronger than most hormones, and it can send you down a moody path when it's unbal-anced. The danger comes when it's imitated by this toxic chemical, which increases its numbers when it shouldn't be too busy.

You Smell Bad

This is a hard pill to swallow, but sometimes, our bodies

and breath smell like the behind of a cow. Foul-smelling breath, stools, or sweat are signs that the liver and colon aren't functioning as they should anymore. They need to detoxify the body and can't handle the load anymore.

You Spend Hours in the Toilet

Constipation is a sign that your body is also toxic. You need to have at least one bowel movement daily, or your cells will absorb the toxins your body's trying to excrete. Constipation is easily solved with more water and fiber.

Your Muscles Ache for No Reason

Keep the inflammation and pain responses in mind to understand where unexplainable aches and pains come from. Your immune system and the bacteria intended to detoxify your body are so busy attacking the places where toxins are overloaded that you feel pain in your muscles.

Your Skin Tells a Story

You know that the liver won't handle too many toxins, and your skin starts to expel toxins through your pores. Now, you can suffer from acne, eczema, blocked pores, and even excessive sweat.

Your Sense of Smell is Whacky

The liver must process toxins found in perfumes and scents. Taking a whiff of your favorite perfume and becoming sick is a sign that toxicity is high. Being nauseated for no reason by someone else's scent is also a sign. Your toxic levels can even be exposed when you get sick after smelling certain foods.

You Have Frequent Digestive Issues

Don't brush frequent digestive problems off as stomach bugs. No one gets stomach bugs five times a month. Diarrhea, vomiting, and stomach contractions are also signs of toxicity if you experience them often like people with IBD and IBS do.

These are signs people often overlook, but you could also be experiencing heart palpitations, shortness of breath, sudden ulcer formations, and emotional instability. Don't forget that numbness, tingling, and tremors signal that something's wrong inside of your body. Your body will always raise the red flag when something isn't right. Listen to the warnings that it sends you, and commit to changing your lifestyle for genuine improvements.

Beware the Toxins That Hide in Plain Sight

The list of toxins we consume is greater than you can imagine because science and the food industry will always try to improve our supply to match the demand. Genetically-modified foods (GMOs) also pose a concern. Science has advanced to the point where our beef is grown from stem cells in a laboratory now. Obviously, not all of it, but how long will it be until our cattle run dry and our mouths still need food? Anyway, some wheat is also being genetically modified now in a process called hybridization (Anderson & Burakoff, 2020).

This means that scientists are targeting specific genes and encouraging them reproduce, especially in wheat products. Eventually, the visible construct of wheat changes over time. Gluten is a natural protein found in wheat, grains, barley, and rye. Wheat already contains more gluten than other products, and the fact that pesticides are being used to speed up the harvesting process is the reason why gluten numbers have peaked in our daily products. The pesticides activate the bacteria that already exist in the crops, and gluten is multiplied.

Just as with anything in life, balanced amounts of gluten are fine for most people; however, excessive amounts lead to gluten intolerance and even Celiac Disease. People with Celiac Disease have an autoimmune disorder where the immune system attacks gluten like a foreign invader. The immune system's response can break down the gut bacteria and cause complete hormonal imbalances. Often, gluten intolerance shows when you're bloated, constipated, tired, or suffer from depression after eating large amounts of it. Gluten is a toxin in excessive numbers. The damage it does to your stomach and intestinal lining can kill the bacteria that is meant to collect nutrients, vitamins, and it can even cause anemia.

It's a good idea to test yourself for gluten intolerance because this chemical found in food, whether modified or not, can become toxic. The majority of your toxins come from food with all the preservatives, additives, chemicals, and pesticides that harm your gut health. However, toxins aren't only present in the food you consume. Personal care products like shampoo, soap, and cream also contain substances that affect your balance. Even toothpaste, body wash, and deodorant contain chemicals. Use natural products instead that haven't been chemicalized to the moon and back.

Environmental factors can also increase toxicity, such as household cleaning agents, pollution, and having no fresh air circulating in your home. Your best chance of being healthy means that you need to limit your exposure to these harmful chemicals. Keep drinking between eight and 10 glasses of water daily to help the body flush the toxins out.

Adding a filter to your kitchen taps might improve your chances of avoiding the environmental pollutants and toxins too. Stay away from anything non-organic, and start visiting the farmer's market to purchase single ingredient foods only. Maintain your bowel movements by increasing your fiber intake to keep you regular.

You want to aim for between one and two bowel movements daily. You can also exercise to flush toxins out by increasing your circulation. The faster your blood moves, the faster the toxins get expelled. Watch out for foods containing heavy metals too, such as bread, and stay clear of medication with heavy metals in them. You can also supplement your body with vitamins and nutrients that bind the toxins before it's expelled. You'll need to have an idea of what's causing your toxicity before you do this though. The bottom line is that you must detoxify your body so that the effects of all these harmful, modernized chemicals and toxins don't lead to heart disorders, brain malfunctions, and hormonal fluctuations that put a toddler to shame.

Life was so much simpler when we could pick an apple straight from the tree, even with all its imperfections. Now, the best we can do is limit our exposure to toxins and rid our bodies of accumulating toxicity.

Chapter 3

O kay, now that you're staring at your grocery cabinet with a suspicious glare, squinting your eyes at the cleaning products you use, and opening every window in your home, you're ready to move onto the testing stage. Precision testing is capable of finding underlying toxins, hormonal imbalances, and bacterial influx to help you understand what your body's going through. There are no guessing games as every test is conducted in a lab, and they're called specialty tests. So, lift your chin, and know that any imbalances in your body are merely a few steps away from correction.

A Quick Note

Specialty tests are done when you request them. Many doctors don't understand the problems with toxins, hormonal imbalances, and the gut-brain connection. They'll test you for everything else under the sun first, leading to some astronomical costs. This is what doctors do because they often need to run blood tests to see what medication or supplement you need in your body. They don't always cater to whether the supplement will be absorbed or discarded by the immune system when it notices all these alien invaders in your system. The imbalance in your body is offset organically, and sometimes, you need to counter the problem with holistic or natural remedies as more medication can further upset the balance.

Naturopathic, holistic, and functional experts will normally use a varied approach instead of prescribing a multitude of medications that could only make the problem worse. They also won't try to cover up the pain because pain is an indicator of something, even if it simply means that your bacteria is running low. Antibiotics will only kill bacteria, the good, the bad, and the ugly combined. Most doctors will give you probiotics to counter this, but some of them forget how harmful western medicine can be on our delicate systems. Specialty doctors, naturopaths, and holistic healers will use specialty tests to find out what's upsetting the immune system because almost every symptom you can think of will somehow lead back to the immune system.

The tests are not run in someone's garage or out of some dodgy place. They're called specialty tests because they look even deeper than the run-of-the-mill examinations most doctors do before prescribing a lengthy list of medications. There are numerous tests you can opt for, and you'll only need to find a medical practitioner who does them. Otherwise, see a holistic healer to point you in the right direction. They check metal levels, vitamin deficiencies, nutritional loopholes, the presence of toxins, and the effect of your current medication. The safest way of restoring the natural balance in your body is to use natural methods.

Testing, One, Two, Three... Which One Should You Consider?

The test you choose will depend on the symptoms that you learned about in the previous chapters. No rule says you can't run all the tests either because knowing more gives you the power to eradicate every problem.

Heavy Metal Test

Heavy metals include arsenic, mercury, and lead. You'd be exposed to lead in the environment more than your food, but rice, particularly brown rice, contains arsenic. Mercury is present in some fish, especially the long-living kind, such as swordfish, marlin, and tuna. In rare cases, you might be exposed to toxic levels of copper, zinc, and iron. Metals are good for you in moderation, but arsenic is commonly used to poison people in crazy reality documentaries. Heavy metal toxicity causes numbness, tingling, brain fog, insomnia, and paralysis in some cases.

Non-organic foods and alcohol also cause heavy metal poisoning. Fortunately, there's a test for it. It's formally called the heavy metals panel, and you can test for all six metals or the three more harmful types. A sample of blood, a 24-hour urine test, or in rare cases, hair or nails can be used to detect the metal levels in your body. You'd have to stop eating seafood for 48 hours before testing, but it can determine whether you're toxified or not, and this information will help you manage your intake and exposure of metals. Chelation therapy is available if your levels are through the roof.

Chelation therapy uses ethylene diamine tetraacetic acid to bind the metals so that they can be excreted from your body. However, even lower metal levels need to be managed by limiting your exposure and removing metals from your diet. More serious reasons for requesting a heavy metals panel are shortness of breath, fluid build-up in the lungs, memory loss, brain dysfunction, behavioral changes, and kidney or liver damage. Allow the doctor or holistic healer to translate the results for you because even low levels of metals are suspect.

They don't stay in the blood or urine for long after exposure. Only a professional can tell you how to manage the presence of this toxin properly by looking at your medical history, risk of ongoing exposure, and symptoms to determine if your lifestyle needs more changes. Your age will also factor into the management because the older you get, the higher your count of mercury is naturally.

Food Sensitive Testing

Knowing what your system is sensitive to is one method of keeping the immune system in balance. From milk that makes you gassy to peanuts that make you look like Freddy Kruger; it all comes down to what your immune system can withstand. Okay, people with peanut allergies typically learn the hard way, but many foods cause a sensitivity that makes the immune system react subtly. Remember that the immune system is primarily made up of the bacteria along your skin and inside your gut. Whether your body reacts to certain foods or not, depends on whether the bacteria and enzymes in your digestive system can break the compounds of your food down.

Your body immediately produces proteins and inflammatory agents that target the unwanted compounds in your system if you're allergic to certain foods, causing a full-blown immune reaction. Either way, the immune system doesn't like what you've eaten and will even target harmless compounds because it sees them as threats. Food sensitivity encumbers allergies and intolerances. Everything is housed under its umbrella because it all causes the immune system to react or overreact. Any food you eat that makes you feel the least bit unwell or like the sickest person on earth needs to be tested.

You'll be pricked with a needle on the arm and exposed directly to the compounds of the food you suspect to be intolerable. Blood tests are also used to measure the level of immunoglobulin E (IgE). The IgE shows how much your immune system responds to the food. It's an antibody that forms when certain chemicals, additives, and preservatives enter your system. Avoid prompting for an immunoglobulin G (IgG) test because this one is a little less reliable. These antibodies are often released after eating food, anyway. Food sensitivities cause the immune system to overreact when it shouldn't, leading to low-level inflammation and unnecessary pain.

Stress Hormone Testing for Adrenal Fatigue

Many of these specialty tests require functional practitioners to translate the results correctly. It doesn't help to visit a doctor that doesn't believe in adrenal fatigue. Adrenal insufficiency is accepted by many doctors, but they don't all agree on adrenal fatigue. How can medical experts believe that the adrenal glands can produce too few stress hormones but not too much? That's some black and white thinking right there. Moreover, doctors won't deny that the stress hormones can be overproduced to create anxiety. Adrenal fatigue is real because the stress hormone called cortisol is vastly connected to the immune system (Philp, 2019).

Cortisol needs to keep you alert, but excessive levels of it break down your immune system. Adrenal fatigue will sometimes be masked under the symptoms of brain fog, depression, light-headedness, and having no energy. The test for adrenal fatigue doesn't exist on its own; you must test your stress hormone levels. The first option is to take a salivary cortisol test to measure how much cortisol is in your system. You can use a home test for saliva collection up to six times during the day. There are even home test kits you can buy that test your urine for higher levels of cortisol. Home kits must test your cortisol levels five or six times over 24 hours before taking the result to your chosen practitioner.

Cortisol levels fluctuate throughout the day, and you need to know whether it's in response to genuine stress or whether it's always running high. Similar to pregnancy tests, the first-morning urine is the most important level you want to measure. This measures the cortisol awakening response (CAR), and the result will give your nutritional therapist an idea of what your stress levels are when you wake up. There shouldn't be high levels at this time of the morning. Some home test kits can also measure dehydroepiandrosterone (DHEA), which is another hormone released by the adrenal glands. Having high amounts of both in the morning and at regular intervals during the day is a sign that you have adrenal fatigue.

Blood tests can also expose unhealthy levels of cortisol, including the other hormones released by the adrenal glands. Whichever test you use, the results must be translated by providing your medical history and symptoms to the functional medicine practitioner or registered nutritional therapist because higher cortisol levels can be caused by many factors. Stress is such a large part of life, and that's why we have so many test options. Another one is called the iris contraction test. This one measures pupil dilation which is just another way of seeing how stressed you are. You sit in a dark room and have light reflecting on your pupils. The pupil will either not contract and remain dilated, or it will contract briefly and dilate quickly to its light-adapting position again.

There are so many options to test for adrenal fatigue, but without the right practitioner to assess other factors for stress, the results won't be as reliable. The saliva and urine tests are the most accurate because you can't test multiple times of the day with a blood or iris contraction test. Work with your practitioner and test at home for the best results.

Neurotransmitter Testing

Turning your attention to the neurotransmitters in your brain is one way of finding the source of your unbalanced health. Your brain has billions of neurons that transmit information and chemicals along the communications networks called synapses. Neurotransmitter testing measures the neurotransmitter chemicals passing through the synapses. The neurotransmitters, also called chemical messengers, can stop or run at doses too low or high to sustain optimal health. This test can often find problems even before symptoms set in. Doctors use it to help people understand why they can't lose weight, why certain hormones are deficient, and a plethora of other reasons.

Every nerve cell in your brain has action potential. This is when the nerve ending activates to transmit chemical messages to the next neuron. Norepinephrine is an important neurotransmitter that assists the action potential, and its close cousin is adrenaline. It excites the nerve endings to ensure that chemicals can pass through it. It also regulates blood pressure, moods, and keeps the gut functioning healthily. It synthesizes into adrenaline when you're stressed. Having too much adrenaline causes weight gain, attention problems, high blood pressure, and increased glucose levels.

Gamma-Aminobutyric acid (GABA) is another important facilitator in the communication lines to ensure neurotransmissions continue. You can have too much GABA which induces a sedative state, giving you brain fog with no energy. Low levels of GABA indicate that you have too little adrenaline in your body, and it can cause seizures, insomnia, and moodiness.

Glutamate is another tested neurotransmitter, and it's the most common one in the brain and body. It regulates your moods and motivation, and it has a hand in keeping your calcium and sodium levels stable. Glutamate is a dangerous neurotransmitter when it accumulates because it causes cell calcification that eventually kills the cell. It's the neurotransmitter associated with degenerative disorders and stroke. Low doses can cause insomnia, a lack of energy, and adrenal fatigue. High doses cause mood disorders and excessive adrenal function.

The histamine neurotransmitter is involved in your immune system, sleep cycles, and GI functions too. Too much histamine in your brain is why you have allergic reactions, inflammation, and digestive problems. Low levels also affect digestion and your mood.

Serotonin is another neurotransmitter identified through the test because it inhibits the communications network. It excites and balances the transmissions to regulate body temperature, moods, metabolism, sexual desire, pain modulation, and sleep cycles. Serotonin doesn't only regulate the brain transmissions as it also manages the gastrointestinal tract (GI) and has a role in numerous organs functioning as they should. An imbalanced level of serotonin leads to carbohydrate cravings, migraines, memory problems, blood pressure issues, and depression.

Dopamine is another neurotransmitter the test looks for. It enhances the transmissions itself and is known as the natural pleasure drug, but it has many other jobs. It strengthens the networks and their surrounding myelin coats, leading to sharper focus, better memory consolidation, and balanced behavior. Dopamine helps the immune system, endocrine system, and GI tract maintain their health. Low levels of dopamine are seen in Parkinson's disease, people with behavioral problems, and addiction. Higher levels of dopamine sustain muscular strength and prevent tremors too.

Creatinine is the final neurotransmitter that's disposed of through your urine. The levels of creatinine in your urine can determine how balanced all the other neurotransmitters are. There are no conditions that can impact the creatinine levels in your urine, even if your kidneys are malfunctioning.

That's why a neurotransmitter test is conducted by sampling your urine to see if all the role players are running at high, balanced, or low levels. Anyone with gastrointestinal problems is advised to have this test done. It can expose hormonal imbalances, adrenal dysfunction, malnourishment, mood stability, brain fog, insomnia, food sensitivities, and thyroid disorders. It can also show problems with chronic pain syndromes, blood pressure issues, glucose instability, migraines, IBS, and autoimmune disorders. It's an all-round test to check everything.

Genetic Mapping

This type of test maps the molecules, proteins, and chromosomes in your body to see if there are any abnormalities. Molecular versions of the test will use your blood to determine if any abnormalities exist in your single deoxyribonucleic acid (DNA) strands, and this exposes genetically predispositions to any conditions. Your functional practitioner will then design a plan for you to use as a guideline to prevent the disorder.

Chromosomal genetic testing is where they take blood to determine whether there are any abnormalities in the longer strand DNA. Looking at the bigger picture is certainly the better way to see if there are any copies of the abnormal gene. Biochemical genetic tests will determine how much protein is in your DNA because excessive amounts of protein are a sign that there's an abnormality. A geneticist will conduct one of the three tests you opt for.

This one doesn't really test for current lifestyle choices, but it identifies problems in your genes that could lead to disorders later in life, allowing you to lead a healthy lifestyle to minimize the risk of developing predisposed disorders. It can also determine whether you're more sensitive to certain toxins from the environment.

Environmental Toxins Test

Environmental toxins can prevent you from losing weight, lead to multiple inflammatory symptoms, and cause food or environmental sensitivities. Your functional practitioner will screen you first to understand what your lifestyle entails because this shows them the root cause of what makes you unwell. Toxins highlighted by this screening can help your practitioner determine what treatment you need, or what lifestyle changes will benefit you. It's recommended to do the environmental toxins test with the heavy metals and food additive panels. There are three kinds of tests available for this one.

The wheat zoom test will require urine to test for antibodies against wheat compounds. It includes gluten and non-gluten components, and antibodies will show the practitioner if your gut is susceptible to these toxins.

The gut wall test requires a stool sample for analysis. Your practitioner must know the integrity of the gut wall that controls the immune system. Stool samples show how healthy your microbiome is. Any imbalances in the microbiome will indicate autoimmune disorders, GI problems, and inflammatory conditions. This test will also show your risk for IBS, IBD, liver disease, metabolic health, nutritional well-being, and cardiovascular health. It looks for 67 kinds of bad bacteria, parasites, viruses, and fungi. The gut wall test also checks for cholic acid, bile acid, pancreatic elastase, and valeric acid. I know this all sounds Greek to you, but the gut wall test is the most comprehensive kind to identify any imbalance that starts in the microbiome.

The third type of environmental toxins test is called a neuronal zoom examination that tests the antibodies of 16 well-known balance disruptors in the brain. The neuronal test is combined with genetic testing to see a larger picture. This is an option for people with brain fog, muscle weakness, and unexplained pain.

This wraps up the myriad of tests available for you to find out why your body is toxic. There are other simple options offered by most practitioners, such as blood and urine tests to see how your hormones fluctuate, but they aren't as comprehensive as the specialty toxin tests. The tests mentioned in this chapter are holistic, naturopathic, and require specialist practitioners, but they look specifically for toxicity. You'll find someone who can help you go through the tests you choose. Knowing the results of your body's toxicity will help you design a lifestyle that prevents further damage and promotes better health.

GETTING YOUR CLEAN STATE KICK-START

Chapter 4

Living healthily starts by removing all the toxins you've encountered before you can dive into the ocean of well-being. Fortunately, there are natural methods of removing the toxins, and you can start with a clean slate again. You'll learn about the dos and don'ts of cleansing your body from toxins, as well as doing it right so that you don't end up back where you are now. Some substitutions and simple detox cleanses can pave the way for you to be as healthy as desired.

Doing It the Right Way

There are so many detoxes available, and you've probably tried a few before if you intended to lose weight or change your well-being. Sadly, there are a few detox suggestions that harm you more than they help you. Some cleanses can also backfire, leaving you quite disappointed. Not everyone will succeed with the same cleanse because we haven't all become toxic the same way. You'll have to learn what works best for you, and having your toxin testing results will help you know what needs to be done. Use the five rules of doing it right and your cleanse won't be fruitless.

Rule number one says that you should only cleanse if it works for you. Don't be part of the trending diets and peer pressure. Some people feel amazing during detoxes and others become agitated, moody, constipated, and exhausted. Some detoxes are strict and immediately deprive your body of everything it loves. This can cause cravings to hit you hard. Your body needs to react positively to cleansing, otherwise, you can simply start living healthy to slowly get rid of the toxins.

This leads to rule number two. Not everyone succeeds in the same detox. The definitions are vast, and you need to choose one that won't make your body retaliate. For some, detox is an abrupt halt to food where it's replaced with juices and smoothies. For others, detox could mean cutting back on all the harmful stuff you once ate. The removal of alcohol, sugar, bread, flour, wheat, and non-organic grains already starts the cleansing process slowly. Toxic fruit and vegetables can be alternated with organic produce.

Rule number three tells you to pause your exercise while you're on a cleanse. Your body is already consuming less of what it normally uses for fuel, and adding strenuous exercise regimes to this is a recipe for disaster. You could lose muscle mass that makes you more prone to injuries, and your metabolism will slow down. That's the opposite of what you're trying to achieve anyway. Detoxes must remove toxins and speed your metabolism up.

Rule number four tells you to use your detox as a gateway into a wholesome lifestyle. Cleanses can make you feel so much better. Your mood changes when it's working, and you can even lose a few pounds and inches. This even adds motivation to continue the lifestyle. A working detox will subside your cravings for salt, sugar, and fatty foods quickly, leaving you with a higher appreciation for whole foods again. You'll also be able to connect faster with your hunger and satisfaction cues after a simple cleanse. Don't allow your detox to go down the drain by eating regular fatty and unhealthy foods as soon as you've dropped three pounds.

The final rule states that a detox diet must never be used as a seesaw. Detoxes are not purging fix-ups. Don't overindulge and come back to your detox after eating 50 hamburgers and three slices of cake over the weekend. Your body can't sustain health if you're moving back and forth between healthy and unhealthy eating. Some people use detoxes like others use excessive exercise, purging, and unhealthy amounts of stool looseners to try to rid the body of toxins after a weekend of fun. This is dangerous behavior and is classed the same as being bulimic. It affects your mental health, and your hormones will become more whacky than ever before. Please seek help if you feel that you've been using the seesaw method of detoxing.

Chiropractic Supercharge

Chiropractors are the last thing on your mind when you think of detoxification. Doctor Daniel Farkas has a surprising method for you to cleanse your body and jumpstart your immune system (Back to Health Chiropractic Center, 2020). Farkas is a chiropractor and functional medicine practitioner in Michigan. He uses his holistic methods to supercharge people's immune systems, removing the risk of future problems and even viruses. Farkas refers to the Spanish Flu in 1918 that took over 600,000 American lives to help you understand how the adjustment of your spine can amplify your immune response.

People in Iowa relied on the traditional medical approach that saw a survival rate of 93.3%, whereas chiropractic healing led to a survival rate of 99.87%. New York's traditional survival rates were 90.9%, and chiropractic results showed a survival rate of

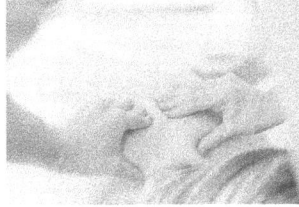

Chiropractor

99.75%. It doesn't seem like much, but it remains a difference. Chiropractors focus on the controls of your health, whether this is toxins, germs, bacteria, or anything that the immune system should pick up as invaders. It enhances your immune system so that your response time to toxic invaders is lessened.

Everyone thinks of chiropractors as practitioners who fix back and neck pain, but they do much more. They also developed more healing techniques than what they used during the Spanish Flu. They work with maps that show the circuitry between the brain and organs in the body. Every gland is connected to the spinal column that runs through to the brain with countless nerves. Your immune system, thyroids, adrenal glands, liver, kidneys, and every gland you can name is linked to the brain through this intricate system. The signals or chemicals that travel through the nerves and into each gland is how the brain instructs the body to erase toxins, and this is the immune system.

Sometimes, we have pinched nerves along the spine that can stop an organ from signaling the brain because communications can't pass through a closed nerve. It works the same way in reverse. How can your brain activate the immune response to an injured or toxic region if the nerve is shut between two spinal discs? Therefore, you must consider a chiropractic approach to make sure your detox won't be fruitless either. Chiropractors are the only medical experts who can identify and adjust the tiny nerve blockages along the spine. They'll then apply pressure and adjust the nerve to move, opening the flow through it again.

Having no closed circuits in your internal communications system is how you start your cleanse. Fortunately, chiropractors have handheld devices to help them find the "short-circuits" today. This handheld device can also be used safely to resonate with pulses that help the practitioner adjust the nerve. Using chiropractic approaches frequently will give you a clean slate of health before you dive into cleanses. The secret is to keep adjusting your spine so that every nerve is free, and that's how the immune system can be ready for any alien toxins.

Full Cellular Cleanse (The Comprehensive Detox)

Toxins are latched onto your cells throughout the body, and you need to remove them from the source. The problem starts and must end in the cells if you want to detox for overall well-being. Cells are capable of regenerating themselves, so cleansing them can help the body get back to its regular self-healing process. It helps you live longer, be healthier, and have a more fulfilling life. You start detoxing the downstream cells, such as the liver, kidneys, and gut to improve every cell along the network. Then you must open the pathways to the upstream cells.

Finally, you enhance the cells in your brain to make an all-round cleanse happen. Having your downstream cells ready will ensure that your brain can rid itself of the toxins without them getting stuck in tissue on the way out. This detox doesn't happen overnight, but it targets the very cells that need to restore themselves, and it keeps your immune system in the best health. Focusing on the cells isn't as simple as a foot bath or colon cleanse alone because these downstream cleanses don't work on the upstream pathways.

You need to change the way you eat and the products you expose yourself to for the recommended times, and add recommendations to support each system. Follow the three phases of the cellular detox. You can also purchase the systemic supplements recommended by Doctor Nick Zyrowski in his 90-day True Cellular Cleanse package (Zyrowski, n.d.). You'll receive a package of sachets to dilute daily to support each cellular change. Make sure you're drinking enough water while taking the supplements.

Preparation Phase: Apply the Five Principles

Prepare your entire system with the five principles by eating healthy, unprocessed, natural foods. Optionally, add the cleanse sachets to improve your cellular preparation. This phase lasts for 30 days.

Principal One

Remove all of the sources of your toxins. The tests have given you an idea of what needs to go. Don't wait until Monday, because every detox or diet starts next week. Throw away all the toxic products, food, and chemicals in your home. Your detox begins slowly and naturally once all toxins are removed.

Principal Two

Allow the cell membranes to regenerate. This is the intelligence of the cell as it collects nutrients and regulates the hormones or chemicals that pass through it. Stick to your whole foods, and use the membrane enhancers found in the cleanse package. Eating healthy fats also promotes cellular regeneration.

Principal Three

Restore energy to the cell's mitochondria. It's the part of your cell that collects nutrients and recycles them into energy to allow the cell to regenerate or detox. You can't open the pathways in phase two without enough cellular energy. The sachets in the package will restore your mitochondria, or avoiding the simple carbs that leave the cells without proper energy will work, too. Only complex carbs must be eaten, which you'll learn more about.

Principal Four

Cellular inflammation is what's causing chronic ailments, and this must be reduced. The membranes become inflamed, and they can't cycle nutrients to avoid genetic weakness. Cellular detox reduces the inflammation and allows the cells to communicate effectively. Eating leafy greens, tomatoes, and olive oil help with this, or the methylation donor and microbiome colonizers from the sachets will work, too. You want to drop sugars, grains, and unhealthy fats from your daily intake.

Principal Five

Finally, you'll be re-establishing methylation, which is a biological process that helps cells repair themselves, detox, fight infections, and communicate effectively (Pompa, 2015). Your body can't sustain health or remove toxic waste from your cells without methylation. Methyl groups regulate stress hormones, turning them on and off to prevent degeneration. Keeping your food toxin-free and using the optional sachets will improve this.

All the principals will establish themselves through clean eating with natural and whole foods, and the cleanse package can help you promote the principles further. You don't need the package, but it helps if you want to ensure deep cleaning to prepare the body and brain.

Body Phase: Supporting and Opening the Pathways

The second part of your detox will continue for another 30 days, and it's called the body phase. Your pathways are stronger after the initial month, so you can now use colon cleanses, supplements recommended by your functional practitioner, and kidney flushes. You're focusing on your downstream body first to make sure your kidneys, liver, colon, and gut are capable of removing the toxins coming from the brain in the last phase. The downstream pathways are called the lymphatic system.

These cells remove toxins from the tissue and push them into the bloodstream. These toxins are then carried to organs that must dispose of them. The majority of your lymphatic cells are in the gut, and that's why you must maintain your new lifestyle after detoxing. You'll be eating healthy now, but you'll also drink lots of water to flush the kidneys. This prevents toxins from flowing through your bloodstream and latching onto new cells. Avoid too much protein in this phase and eat potassium-rich foods, such as yogurt and citrus.

Use whey water as it contains potassium to support the kidneys further. Staying hydrated is one way of flushing the toxins from your body. Use a coffee enema to open and support the liver because bile is filled with toxins. Bile acts as digestive fluids, so you need to keep it clean. It also collects nutrients for the cells. Coffee enemas, milk thistle, leafy greens, and dandelion tea remove the excess bile before the toxicity escalates. Opening and supporting your gut matters during the body phase, too. Intermittent fasting, whey water, purified water, or broth made from grass-fed cow bones will work for the gut.

You must avoid toxic foods that stop the cellular pathways from opening. You should be supporting them by avoiding sugar, GMOs, and grains. Make sure you're getting enough of what your body needs to restore the cells. Vitamin D, K1, K2, B12, iodine, and magnesium are good supporting supplements. You can also use a multivitamin to keep your cells sustained with nutrients. Become active during this phase, sleep better, and learn relaxation techniques. Leading a clean lifestyle is going to restore the cells in the brain, too, but that comes next.

When the brain cells start ridding themselves of toxins, your downstream system is ready to remove them from your body. The cleanse package will contain the same ingredients as the first phase, but there will also be a binder now. The binding agent latches onto toxins and binds them before they can re-enter the system. It's recommended to start using a binding agent in the second phase. Look for a binding agent at the drugstore if you're unsure. It should contain activated carbon, baozene, and bacillus coagulans to ensure proper binding. One brand is called *Bind*, which acts as a multi-binder to remove metals and toxins.

Use binding agents on the on-off cycle. Take them for four to seven days, and then leave them for seven to 10 days. *CytoDetox* is another good brand because it fights through inflammation to get inside the membrane of the cells.

Discuss a binding agent with a functional practitioner if you're uncertain.

Brain Phase: Cleaning Grey Matter

The brain is a sensitive organ and needs to be detoxed for another 30 days after the other phases are complete. Now, the neurotoxins in the brain can move through the body and be excreted by the healthier cells downstream. Maintain your new lifestyle with the five principals in phase one. Don't return to eating processed, non-organic, and toxic foods stuffed with the wrong chemicals. The Zybrowski cleanse package will help your brain rid itself of the neurotoxins through the open pathways. Otherwise, you can supplement your new lifestyle with a few natural remedies.

Continue using the on-off strategy with your binding agent for this phase, but add alpha-lipoic acid that also contains biotin. This encourages the brain to renew abnormal cells. Speak to your functional practitioner about any supplements you want to use. The bottom line of every phase is healthy eating, but you can add enhancers by choice. Try to continue taking a methylation donor with a few vitamins you need. Taking a multi-mineral supplement is also advised now. Minerals keep the electrolytes balanced in your body while your brain is restoring its cells.

The five principals in this detox will be covered in the lifestyle changes in the coming chapters. Sometimes, making simple changes can make a huge difference, but use the supplements and phases to detox slowly. It starts by preparing the body and mind, opening the gateway through your liver and kidneys, and finally, allowing the brain to remove neurotoxins through the open stream with binding agents and mineral supplements. Ninety-days seems like a long time, but it's the start of the rest of your life.

The Abrupt Master Cleanse

A master cleanse is used if you want to jump start your cleanse. It's so abrupt that it's recommended to ease into it first. The body won't do well with a liquid detox if you don't introduce it slowly. Ease into over five days.

Days One and Two: Cut all the toxins from your diet, including alcohol, processed foods, sugar, dairy, meat, and caffeine. Replace them with whole, raw foods, such as organic veggies and fruit.

Day Three: Make smoothies to get yourself used to liquid food. Why not add some soup, broths, or freshly squeezed fruit juice?

Day Four: Cut down further by only drinking freshly-squeezed orange juice and water. Add some maple syrup to your juice for added calories, and have one laxative type tea before bed. Any tea that makes your stomach regular will work.

Day Five: Apply the master cleanse now.

Most of your calories are going to come from a home-brew now. Use two tablespoons of freshly-squeezed lemon juice, two tablespoons of pure maple syrup, a fifth of a teaspoon of cayenne pepper (or more if you like the taste), and eight to 12 ounces of purified water. Mix all the ingredients, and drink at least six portions daily. You can have another portion if you feel hungry. You're also welcome to use herbal laxatives before bed or warm saltwater in the morning to keep your stomach regular. Depending on how long you can last, continue from day five until you've been on the cleanse for between 10 and 40 days.

You'll also need to ease out of the cleanse slowly.

Day One: Replace your cleanse cocktail with fresh orange juice.

Day Two: Add some vegetable soup today.

Day Three: Feel free to have some organic fruit and vegetables.

Day Four: You should be eating normally by day four, keeping in mind that all your food is now organic and unprocessed.

The master cleanse can reduce inflammation, aid in weight loss, and remove toxins from your body.

You have two incredible options to detox yourself, but remember that applying a wholesome lifestyle will also detox your system in time. The rules never waiver because you aren't detoxing if you aren't coping with it.

THE NUTRITIONAL SIDE OF A GOOD LIFE

Chapter 5

Clean eating is a term often used, but understanding what it does for you, and how many options you have is another ballgame. Learning to eat clean is like taking a step back to when food was simpler, healthier, and didn't contain all the junk it does today. Nothing is boring or stagnant about eating clean, either. There's a wide variety of options to make the most incredible meals. You're about to learn the secrets to clean eating and cutting back on all the junk that puts your health at risk.

What Is Clean Eating?

The first golden rule of eating clean is to remove all toxic, processed, packaged, and non-organic foods from your life. You want real foods that maximize your nutritional intake with every bite. The word 'natural' is important because you want food that's as close to its natural state as you can find it. You don't want food sprayed with chemicals, processed to prolong the shelf life, or grown in a lab. You also want to cut all the ingredients that have become so refined that it can take a buffalo down. There are so many natural foods that provide the nutrients our body craves.

Clean eating removes all the processed fats, mountains of salt, and oceans of sugar. People didn't need all the modifications to their foods a few decades back, so why must you live with chemicals you can't even pronounce in your food? It should take you more than 60 seconds to make your food, too. Anything that reheats in 60 seconds is unnatural. Salads, organic fruit, and raw vegetables are the only instant clean foods you should eat. Your main goal remains to enhance your health. Remove all the toxic waste from your home and consumption, and replace it with food that truly benefits your entire body and mind.

Clean eating is part of an entire lifestyle and doesn't mean that you'll be eating raw carrots either unless you want to. You can do so much with the ingredients recommended, and leading a clean lifestyle means that you won't be removing every carb and enjoyable food either. The longer you're committed to clean eating, the more you'll experience the benefits, and you won't want to return to your old ways again.

Priceless Clean Changes

The thought of clean eating can be overwhelming for anyone who still thinks it's a diet. It has nothing to do with dieting, but there are some great guidelines to remove what harms you, and replace it with food that promotes health and longevity.

Long-Term Goals

Enter the journey as a long-running lifestyle change. You don't have to drop everything at once and scare yourself into the arms of candy and ice-cream. Slow and steady is the best option while you're finding your feet. Don't start weighing your food, rather make small changes without cutting everything you love at once. Unfortunately, the diet mentality of all or nothing often frightens people back to unhealthy eating.

Varying Definitions

Healthy eating isn't the same for everyone because you might be a vegetarian, but your friend might love fasting instead. Don't forget rule number one. You must learn what works for you and what you love. Don't expect your plate to look the same as someone else's.

Take it Easy

Go easy on yourself if you eat the wrong thing. Remember that this is a long-term commitment, so there's no rush to the finish line. The finish line doesn't exist.

Know Why You're Doing This

Recognize why you're changing your lifestyle. Are you doing it to become healthier, live longer, or lose weight? Or, are you doing it to please loved ones who always tell you to eat better? No, you must only be doing this for yourself. You must *want* to eat clean. You can't do it for anyone else. Your thoughts can also be toxic, so it doesn't matter if you're stocking your fridge with whole foods if you're telling yourself that you need to get healthy because of what someone else said.

Cook at Home

Start cooking your meals at home more frequently. It's so much easier to keep track of what you're consuming if you're making it from scratch. You don't know what toxins exist in restaurants or takeout food.

Experiment With Same Seasons

Many people don't know this, but you can experiment with your foods if you just allow your mind to be more curious. Foods that grow in the same season tend to complement each other well. Be the chef who throws a bunch of stuff together and makes something incredibly original. Summer fruits make amazing salads together, but winter fruits make great smoothies when liquified. Surprise yourself with new concoctions.

Quality Over Calories

Focus on the quality of your food more than the calories you're eating. Your brain will resist if you keep cooking food that meets the calorie standards, but it tastes like something that fell off the farmer's wagon and rolled in the dirt.

Read Those Labels!

Be aware of everything you use by reading labels. Remember that your single-ingredient labels are the clean foods that haven't been processed extensively. However, you can commit to five ingredients or less. You must be able to recognize, read, and pronounce the ingredients on the label. There should be no added fats, sugars, or salt. Be careful of preservatives in bottled and canned products, too.

Even roasted nuts have been burned in unhealthy vegetable oils. Salad dressing is a problem, too, because it might be easier to pour it on your salad, but it's cleaner to make it from scratch. Clean eating means less packaged products, but you can't avoid all of them. Some vegetables, nuts, and meat will be packaged, so read the labels.

Processed Foods Go in the Bin!

Stay away from processed foods as every ingredient that

doesn't come straight from the field is slightly to highly processed. You don't need to panic about slightly processed food that requires some mechanical processing or that which has been packaged lightly if you can still read the ingredients. Frankenfoods are highly processed foods made in factories, grown in labs, and sprayed with gallons of pesticides. Their colors might be brighter, but that's only because they've been enhanced chemically.

Your taste buds become bombarded with flavor enhancers, and you'll only crave more salt, sugar, and fats. Take baby steps out of highly processed food to give your taste buds a chance to gather their bearings again. Whole foods seem tasteless at first because your taste buds have been poisoned. Slowly introduce yourself to whole foods again to learn to appreciate the natural flavors when your taste buds readjust themselves. You'll be surprised what a natural spice and herb shelf can do to food.

Processed food is an unnatural, unhealthy, and disease-stimulating option. They've been mutilated to where the compounds put you at a higher risk of inflammation and atherogenics, which are fatty plaques that stick to the artery walls leading to your heart. A systematic review conducted by University Nacional de Córdoba in Argentina confirmed that the excessive fatty plaque in the arteries caused by processed food is to blame for the increasing rates of heart disease (Defagó et al., 2014). Save your heart by throwing processed food in the bin.

Artificial Flavorings Are for Artificial Beings

Stay away from the so-called fat-free, sugar-free choices because they contain endless traces of artificial flavor enhancers. Don't be fooled by the artificial sweeteners and flavorings that make your brain crave more because they release all the feel-good chemicals. Food companies will throw anything into their "secret recipes" to make you addicted to their junk.

Prep Your Meals

Meal prepping is the savior of anyone who doesn't want to cook five times in two days. Experiment with recipes you can cook once and eat three times. For example, you can make a quinoa salad with free-range chicken breast, and keep it in the fridge for two days. Meal prepping also helps you have options when you arrive home with an appetite of a lion. If your salad is ready, and it's soaked up all the goodness from standing overnight, you're going to eat it immediately.

Listen to Your Hunger Cues

Let your hunger guide you, and never allow it to be overwhelmed. The hungrier you are, the more your brain will crave things it shouldn't. Always eat when you're hungry. Forget the clock, and throw the diet plan away. Your body is the only thing guiding your food intake. It will send you signals to say: "Hey! I'm hungry!" Don't let your body reach the starving stage.

Keep the Environment Clean

Create a healthy eating environment, too. Try to avoid environments that aren't conducive to your clean eating. It's hard to sit between friends at an Italian restaurant when their plates are stacked with lasagna, and you're ordering a salad. In rare cases, you can absorb mental nourishment from your friends and eat something Italian with them if you're not doing it often. Otherwise, try to control the environment where you're eating and the people surrounding you.

Add Organic Fruit and Vegetables

Fruit and vegetables aren't the enemies; it's the pesti-cides, processing, and packaging that makes them unhealthy. Raw fruit and vegetables are loaded with vita-mins, nutrients, minerals, fiber, and compounds that keep your inflammation under control. Harvard Medical School conducted studies to identify the impact of eating organic fruit and vegetables (Farvid et al., 2016). Harvard's purpose was to see if the biological compounds could make a differ-ence in women who were genetically at risk for breast cancer.

More than 90,000 women between the ages of 27 and 44 participated in getting an accurate understanding of the effi-ciency of the anti-inflammatory agents and antioxidants found in fruit and vegetables, and how they keep your cells balanced to prevent abnormalities. They also keep your chemical transmissions under check, and this helps the immune system work correctly. The nutritional value of organic fruit and vegetables far outweighs the pathogens in the body, lowering the risk of cancer.

Fruit and vegetables are the perfect additives for clean eating because you can pick them straight from the bush, wash them, and eat them raw. Using these ingredients is simple with three rules.

1. Color your salads with at least three options that aren't green.
2. Berries, orange slices, and chopped apples go with any meal.
3. Always wash veggies, and toss them with olive oil to keep in a container in the fridge for easy access.

Introduce Complex Carbs (For Better Sleep Too)

Refined carbohydrates are the worst choice, and they don't define clean eating. Simple carbs are connected to inflammation, fatty liver, obesity, and insulin resistance. They're found in white bread, ready-to-eat cereals, oats, and refined grains. Complex carbs are better, and they're found in less processed foods like brown rice, quinoa, sweet potato, sprouted grain bread, some vegetables, and steel-cut oats. Complex carbs take longer to break down, and they keep you satisfied between meals.

They also help you sleep better at night because food that balances your glucose levels and keeps cortisol at bay helps you sleep better. Whole, unrefined grains are also sources of complex carbs, and they pack a punch of nutrients and fiber that whammies your system into better health. Best of all is that those complex carbs are food for the gut bacteria and help to maintain gut health. So, never cut carbs, but only cut simple and refined carbs.

Avoid the Easy Fats

Spreads and oils are unhealthy and processed to a point you can't recognize. Vegetable oil and margarine *aren't* clean options. Avoid those omega-6 fats in your clean diet. Omega-6 increases inflammation, leading to a higher risk of heart disease and obesity. Artificial trans fats were actually banned in America, but some margarine still contains trace amounts of it. Sandwich spreads are just as processed and unhealthy. Avoid all bad fats and replace them with extra virgin olive oil, butter, raw nuts, omega-3 fish, and avocado.

Added Sugar Is a No!

You can't believe where they put added sugar today. Condiments and sauces have oodles of sugar, even if they don't taste sweet. Table sugar is enemy number one, but high-fructose corn syrup is enemy number two. High levels of fructose were matched to fatty liver disease, obesity, heart disease, diabetes, and cancer (Spritzler, 2019). Small amounts of honey and maple syrup are the better options for eating clean, but not if you're diabetic or have metabolic syndrome.

Choose Your Drinks

Water should always be the first choice because it keeps the brain and body hydrated enough to function as it should. Alcohol should be limited as much as possible. It's fermented vegetables, grains, and yeast. Wine isn't the worst option, but not if you're having it every day. Alcohol causes inflammation, digestive issues, and affects the liver. There are several diseases blamed on alcohol consumption, but once the liver fails, the body cannot excrete toxins anymore. Limit or remove alcohol from your consumption.

Learn the Value of Vegetable Substitutions

Cauliflower is one of the most versatile vegetables that can be a substitute for pizza dough, flour, rice, and mash. Spaghetti squash replaces pasta, and zucchini is great for a noodle substitution. Unless you try them, you won't know how tasty they are.

Steer Clear of Packaged Snacks

Muffins, granola bars, and crackers are processed snacks. Stick to healthier and raw options by making sure you always have fruit on hand or making the products from scratch with gluten-free, organic, pesticide-free wheat and flour products.

Choose Ethical Animal Products

Don't buy meat that isn't organic anymore. You don't want to see what the factory farming animals live through. The conditions alone are frightening. These animals are also pumped with steroids to speed growth and antibiotics to fight the inevitable infections surrounding them in the disgusting environment. They also get injected with testosterone and estrogen to further enhance their growth. Grass-fed beef is the highest in omega-3 anti-inflammatory agents and antioxidants. Stop buying grain-fed animal products. Your dairy, meat, chicken, and eggs must come from ethically-raised animals.

Stay Away From Gluten

Gluten isn't going to help your journey, so start reading the labels to know where your wheat and grain products come from before stocking your pantry. You want natural, organic, and chemical-free products only. You've learned about the disgrace of gluten, and what it does to your body. Give your body a chance to regenerate by avoiding gluten that leads to Celiac Disease.

Clean eating has a myriad of options, and you can start implementing the options as you feel comfortable. Some of them won't even make a difference to your idea of food, but throwing the processed and easy foods away might seem challenging. Do it at your pace because the first rule of eating clean is to know that this is a life-long commitment.

Glorious Herbs

Herbs have been around as long as humans have, and they bring us some amazing remedies that could boost your clean eating (Dog, 2014). Ancient cultures still use herbs to fight viruses, infections, and chronic disorders today. Even western medicine has added chamomile to over-the-counter calmatives because there's nothing purer, cleaner, and healthier than herbal remedies. You can fight inflammation, toxins, insomnia, and GI disorders. Choose some natural remedies for your new lifestyle.

Ashwagandha

This herb boosts the immune system and reduces inflammation, but don't use it if you have thyroid issues. Steam one teaspoon of dried ashwagandha in hot water, and drink it as a tea twice daily.

Calendula

This is another great option to relieve inflammation in the throat, gut, and mouth. It can also be used as a topical ointment for rash and wounds. Steep two teaspoons of petals in hot water for 10 minutes. Gargle with the strained water or drink it as a tea.

Catnip

Catnip doesn't only make cats happy as it can relieve upset stomachs and reduce your anxiety, too. Steep one teaspoon of dried catnip in a cup of hot water for five minutes, strain it, and drink it as a tea.

Cranberry

Raw and unprocessed cranberry juice can relieve bladder infections and inflamed prostates. Drink half a cup twice daily.

Echinacea

Rarely, some people have allergic reactions, but this herb boosts immune system compounds and fights upper-respiratory viruses. Steep one teaspoon of dried echinacea in a cup of hot water for 10 minutes. Strain it, and drink it up to three times daily.

Garlic

Garlic is a potent killer of bad bacteria in the gut, preventing colds, influenza, and diarrhea. It can also lower blood pressure but isn't advised for people who use blood-thinners like warfarin. Eating one to two fresh cloves daily keeps your microbiome balanced.

Ginger

Ginger also fights stomach problems, such as nausea, vomiting, and diarrhea. It combats colds and flu as well, but pregnant women shouldn't consume too much. One root daily is advised for anyone because it can also upset the stomach if you use too much. Steep one small, fresh root in a cup of hot water, and strain it before drinking it once daily.

Ginseng

This plant helps for physical and mental fatigue. It also improves blood flow and combats colds. Ginseng is often misidentified, so make sure you purchase it from a reliable health store. You'd steep one dried teaspoon and one sliced root in a cup of hot water for 10 minutes before straining it and drinking it once or twice daily.

Hibiscus

This one works for kidney flushes, and it reduces your blood pressure. Use between one and two teaspoons of dried Hibiscus in a cup of hot water. Steep it for 10 minutes, strain it, and drink it twice daily.

Lemon Balm

This herb relieves digestive upset, anxiety, muscle tension, and is a calming sedative. Throw five or six fresh leaves in a hot cup of water and let it steep for five minutes. Strain it, and drink it as many times as you want to.

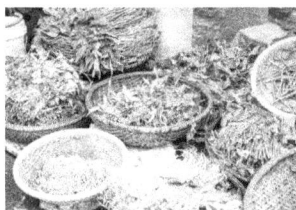

Herbs

Licorice

This is a powerful plant extract that reduces inflammation, restores mucous membranes, and protects or heals the

GI tract. Never use high doses for more than a week because it can raise your blood pressure or steal your potassium. Simmer one freshly sliced root with one dried teaspoon in a hot cup of water for 10 minutes. Strain your tea, and drink it once or twice daily for no more than seven days.

Milk Thistle

This herb protects the liver and kidneys from toxicity. Speak to your functional practitioner about recommending a safe extract and use between 400 and 700 mg divided throughout the day.

Nettle

Nettle is great for relieving allergy symptoms, reducing inflammation around the prostate, and it gives you valuable nutrients. Throw two teaspoons of leaves in a cup of hot water, and steep it for 10 minutes. Drink it up to three times daily.

Thyme

This common kitchen herb is known for replacing good bacteria and removing the bad guys. Steep one dried teaspoon in a cup of hot water for 10 minutes and strain it. Split the cup into three portions for the day.

Herbs can benefit you endlessly. Start introducing some teas with natural remedies into your day to make sure your clean lifestyle is at its peak.

NATURAL FOOD RECIPES AND SAMPLE MENUS TO MAKE YOU DROOL

Chapter 6

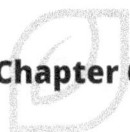

E ating clean is becoming more of a reality than the dream it once was, but you need to be inspired by some great recipes, meal planning, and the idea of superfoods. I'll share a few of my favorite recipes with you and give you a one-week plan so that making the change isn't as challenging as it seems. Brace yourself for the most mind-blowing, mouth-watering, and reality-redefining recipes you'll ever taste. Don't forget that you're encouraged to experiment with new ideas, vegetables, and raw foods, so bring forth your chef toque!

Introducing Superfoods

You know that organic and whole products are best, but did you know that some vegetables can blow the trumpets of healthy living? Some vegetables are superfoods. There are four kinds of vegetables you can use.

Leafy greens are the first-level superfoods of healthy eating. They have little to no carbs, which are complex enough to satisfy your body. Leafy greens are the most jam-packed with nutrients to make your body function at its finest. Dark leafy greens give you nutrients, minerals, and vitamins, such as kale and spinach. Collard greens are also high in fiber. The best is that these greens are all amazing for smoothies, salads, and wraps. Eating them raw is recommended so that you don't lose the nutrients.

Then you have stemmed and flowering veggies, such as spring onions, zucchini, cucumber, asparagus, peas, cauliflower, broccoli, celery, lettuce, green beans, and artichokes. Any vegetables with edible stems or flowers are in this category. These veggies are also superfoods even though they contain slightly higher amounts of carbs. Cooking or steaming some of these second-level superfoods will enhance the nutrients, such as steamed broccoli and cauliflower.

Seeded vegetables are borderline and contain more natural sugars and carbs. The dictionary explains edible plants with seeds as fruit, but bell peppers are known as vegetables. Yellow peppers, green peppers, cherry tomatoes, okra, and jalapenos are seeded veggies.

Finally, starchy vegetables are those we must take caution with. They include sweet potatoes, carrots, onions, squash, beetroot, garlic, and parsnip. Normal potatoes, yams, peas, and legumes should be avoided at all costs as their carb content is too high. Starch is also a fancier word for carbohydrates, but you can use the starchy veggies in this list sparingly.

The chart below shows you how many carbs are found in the vegetables you'd use. The vegetables in the table have been measured as one cup each, keeping in mind that varying weights will fill a cup. The carbs are measured in grams (g).

Vegetable	Carbs	Vegetable	Carbs	Vegetable	Carbs
Spinach	1.1 g	Alfalfa Sprouts	1.2 g	Chard	1.2 g
Bok Choy	1.5 g	Romaine Lettuce	1.5 g	Iceberg Lettuce	1.6 g
Collard Greens	2 g	Mushrooms	3.1 g	Celery	3.3 g
Summer Squash	3.8 g	Cucumbers	3.8 g	Zucchini	4 g
Radishes	4.3 g	Eggplant	4.8 g	Cabbage	5 g
Asparagus	5.2 g	Cauliflower	5.7 g	Broccoli	5.8 g
Red Bell Pepper	5.8 g	Tomatoes	5.8 g	Fennel	6.3 g
Kale	6.7 g	Seaweed	6.7 g	Green Bell Pepper	6.9 g
Okra	7 g	Spaghetti Squash	7 g	Scallions	7.3 g
Snow Peas	7.4 g	Pumpkin	7.5 g	Tomatillos	7.7 g
Bamboo Shoots	7.9 g	Brussel Sprouts	7.9 g	Turnips	8.4 g
Green Beans	9.9 g	Carrots	12.3 g	Leeks	12.6 g
Avocado	12.8 g	Celery Root	14.4 g	Artichokes	18.8 g

Your superfoods are vegetables, but they must be incorporated with their carbohydrate contents in mind. You can't eat starchy vegetables alone and expect to lead a healthy lifestyle. Rather eat higher amounts of healthy fats, which include grass-fed beef, raw nuts, extra virgin olive oil, coconut oil, butter, omega-3 rich fish, and avocado. Try to aim at keeping your carb intake to about 10% of your daily consumption. Your healthy fats shouldn't exceed a total of 25%, and you can allocate the remainder of your intake to protein.

Just keep in mind that all your protein is sourced organically and ethically. Nevertheless, this is about vegetable superfoods because you aren't weighing your food. That would mean that you're on a diet, but hell no, you're not!

Enter the Mouth-Watering Recipes

These are some of my favorite recipes for breakfast, lunch, dinner, and snack times. I don't count calories, rather I live by the clean rules. Every ingredient must be as natural and close to its original state as possible before it enters the pan or blender. Spices must also be natural and herbs are welcome. I use pink Himalayan salt or coarse sea salt minimally. My pepper is also freshly ground. You're welcome to change my recipes as you learn about new ingredients that complement it better for you. Adding more superfoods to your plate is a must. This table will also help you simplify your recipes, rather than measuring everything precisely.

Recipe Conversion Table / Temperatures				
Easy Conversions		**Oven Temperatures**		
A dash	1/16 teaspoon (tsp)	Description	Farhenheit	Gas Levels
A pinch	1/8 tsp	Cool	275	1
2 tablespoons (tbsps)	1 ounce (oz)	Moderate	350	4
1 tablespoon (tbsp)	3 teaspoons (tsps)	Hot	425	7
1 tablespoon	1/2 fluid ounces (fl oz)			
16 tbsp	1 cup			
1 cup	8 fl oz			
1 cup	1/2 pound (lbs)			
1 cup	3 oz - (Dry ingredients)			
4 cups	32 fl oz			
1 lbs - (Meat)	16 oz			
1/2 stick of butter	4 tbsps / 2 oz			
1 stick of butter	8 tbsps / 1/2 cup / 4 oz			

You can't miss with an easy conversion table! I'll use cups and simpler measurements where possible because I don't weigh anything. The oven temperatures have been simplified for gas and electric as well, and you can use the gas setting levels to choose the right stove-top levels for both. Now, we can dive into the recipes!

Flamboyant Egg Salad (Breakfast)

Eggs give you healthy proteins early in the morning. Please ensure that your eggs are free-range. Egg salad might sound boring, but what you throw into it is what spruces it up. A bland idea can turn into something visually attractive and as tasty as it comes. You can also prepare this beforehand. However, don't store it for more than 48 hours in the fridge because boiled eggs have a weird smell.

Serves: Four
Prep Time: 14 minutes
Cooking Time: Nine minutes
Ingredients:

- 1 tsp freshly-squeezed lemon juice
- 1 tsp balsamic vinegar
- 4 tbsps organic mayonnaise
- A dash of Himalayan salt
- Freshly-ground black pepper
- 1 tsp chopped chives
- 1 tsp finely-chopped bell pepper (any color)
- 8 eggs
- 1 cubed avocado
- ¼ cup organic bacon bits
- 4 lettuce leaves
- 2 tbsps sundried tomatoes
- 1 tbsp extra virgin olive oil

Directions:

1. Boil your eggs for nine minutes and peel them.
2. Fry your bacon bits in olive oil on moderate heat until they're crispy.
3. Combine the mayonnaise, chives, salt, pepper, and bell peppers in a medium bowl and whisk them.
4. Chop the boiled eggs up finely and mix them into the mayonnaise concoction.
5. Splash the lemon juice and balsamic vinegar over the avocado.
6. Mix the avocado into the eggs.

7. Place the lettuce leaves on four plates and divide the egg mixture between them.
8. Sprinkle your bacon bits and sundried tomatoes over the four plates and enjoy!

Crazy Smoothie (Breakfast)

The reason I call this a crazy smoothie is that most people wouldn't combine the ingredients that I do, but they have no idea what they're missing. Smoothies are your gateway to being as experimental as Doctor Frankenstein, and there are no limits to what you can throw into them. This smoothie is best consumed immediately, but you can store smoothies in the fridge overnight. Most smoothies don't store well because of the fresh ingredients.

You can use bananas, berries, kiwis, and even leafy green vegetables. Yes, you can throw some kale into your experiments. I love using alternative milk rather than full-dairy cow's milk. Almond milk is a good option if you're not getting milk straight from the cow. Welcome to the crazy smoothie that everyone judges me for.

Serves: Two
Prep Time: Two minutes
Blending Time: Two minutes
Ingredients:

- 1 chopped avocado
- 8 juicy, diced organic strawberries
- 2 tbsps crushed walnuts
- 2 cups almond milk
- 2 tbsps honey

Directions:

1. Throw everything into the blender, including the avocado, strawberries, almond milk, walnuts, and honey.
2. Blend for two minutes.
3. Pour into two glasses and enjoy my crazy mixture.

Fragrant Oats (Breakfast)

This recipe is a secret for anyone who wants to maintain a flat belly. Remember to use organic products, especially the oats. You can also supplement the breakfast with a glass of oat milk that contains no added sugars. The spices will create a homemade pumpkin spice mix so that you don't have to buy the fragrant spice in a processed form.

Serves: Two
Prep Time: 10 minutes
Cooking Time: 20 minutes
Ingredients:

- 3 cups purified water
- 1 cup steel-cut oats
- 2 tbsps olive oil
- ½ tbsp cinnamon
- ½ tsp ground ginger
- ½ tsp ground nutmeg
- ¼ tsp cloves
- 1 tsp raw honey
- 1 chopped apple
- 1 sliced banana
- 1 tbsp pumpkin seeds

Directions:

1. Pour the water into a medium pot and let it boil on a moderate heat.
2. Place the oats and olive oil in a pan, and allow this to toast for two minutes to bring the flavor out.
3. Transfer the oats to the water.
4. Mix all the spices and drop the blend into the water.
5. Add the honey and reduce the stove-top temperature to low.
6. Enjoy the fragrant spices coming from the pot as it cooks for another 18 minutes.
7. Allow the chopped apple to toast in the pan where you had the oats.
8. Combine the apple and oats, and top it with the banana before sprinkling the pumpkin seeds over it.

Snack Attack! Fruit Salad

The best food for snacks is fruit. Eating fruits with high water content also helps you flatten your stomach and stay hydrated. Alter the recipe for the season you're in, and you can always substitute ingredients for what you like. Fruit salads are always best prepared beforehand so that the juices can stir overnight to make the natural sweetness come out.

Serves: Four
Prep Time: Two minutes
Cooking Time: Zero!
Ingredients:

- ½ cup chopped watermelon
- ½ cup finely-chopped mango
- ½ cup halved grapes
- ½ cup diced smooth-skin peaches
- 4 sliced strawberries
- 1 peeled and diced kiwi
- 1 whole orange
- 2 tbsps crushed walnuts
- 2 Drops of Liquid Stevia

Directions:

1. Throw all the fruits except the juiced orange into a medium bowl.
2. Squeeze the orange juice into the bowl and toss the fruit.
3. Sprinkle with the walnuts and Stevia and let the salad stand in the fridge overnight.
4. Divide it into four portions and enjoy!

Quinoa Salad (Lunch)

I love experimenting with quinoa salad because it can also store well in the fridge for up to two days. The list of things you can add is also vaster than you think. Quinoa is a whole grain that doubles as a staple, side dish, salad, or stuffing for wraps. My idea is always to make it colorful when using it for a salad. You can add fruit, vegetables, seeds, and nuts. This salad can also be used as a side dish.

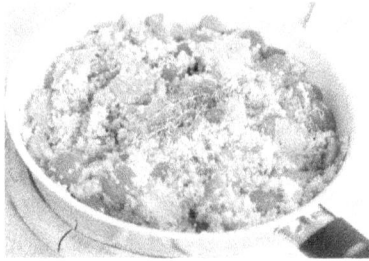

Quinoa Salad Variation

Serves: Four
Prep Time: 10 minutes
Cooking Time: 15 minutes
Ingredients (Salad):

- 2 cups uncooked quinoa
- 1 ½ cups pre-cooked chickpeas (It takes 45 minutes to cook them yourself, but they can be stored in the fridge for later use.)
- 4 cups purified water
- 1 cup diced cucumber
- 2 cups yellow bell pepper chopped finely
- 2 cups diced bok choy
- ½ cup mixed seeds and nuts (sunflower seeds, walnuts, and pine nuts)
- ½ cup sundried tomatoes
- ¼ cup dried cranberries
- 1 cup mixed fresh herbs (chopped cilantro, parsley, and dill)

Ingredients (Homemade Dressing):

- ½ cup olive oil
- ¼ cup balsamic vinegar

- 1 ½ tsps Dijon mustard
- 1 tsp honey
- ½ tsp sea salt
- ½ tsp freshly-ground pepper
- ¼ cup freshly-squeezed lemon juice

Directions:

1. Rinse the quinoa under cold water for 30 seconds.
2. Dry the quinoa in a clean cloth or paper towel.
3. Add the water and quinoa to a pan to cook on high heat to bring it to a boil.
4. Lower the temperature to a low-moderate level and allow it to simmer uncovered for 10 to 15 minutes.
5. Move the pan off the heat and let it stand covered for five minutes.
6. Allow the quinoa to cool down before making the salad.
7. Combine the quinoa with the chickpeas, herbs, bell pepper, cucumber, bok choy, and the nut/seed mixture.
8. Add the dried cranberries and tomatoes and toss the salad.
9. Use a small bowl to whisk together the salt, pepper, lemon juice, olive oil, mustard, vinegar, and honey together.
10. Pour the dressing over the salad and give it a few minutes to absorb the flavors.

Salsa Verde Lamb Kebabs (Lunch or Dinner)

This recipe is amazing, but you must combine it with one of the coming vegetable dishes to fill it with superfoods. The Salsa Verde spice rub will be made from scratch, and the reason I use lamb is that it contains very little fat. The fat is healthy as long as your lamb is organic and ethically-raised.

Serves: Four
Prep Time: 15 minutes
Cooking Time: 10 minutes
Ingredients (Salsa Verde):

- ¼ cup chopped mint
- ½ cup chopped parsley
- 1 oz freshly-filleted anchovies
- 1 tbsp freshly-crushed capers
- 2 tbsps pine nuts
- The zest of 1 lemon
- ½ crushed garlic clove
- 1 tsp freshly-diced chilies
- ½ cup olive oil
- A pinch of sea salt

Ingredients (Lamb Kebabs):

- 10 oz of cubed boneless lamb
- 1 whole eggplant cubed
- A pinch of sea salt and freshly-ground pepper
- 1 freshly-squeezed lemon
- 6 rosemary stems
- 4 tbsps olive oil

Directions:

1. Blend all the Salsa Verde ingredients except for the olive oil and salt together until it's a fine mixture.
2. Add the olive oil slowly to the blender while it's running.
3. Sprinkle the salt and combine to taste.
4. Preheat your oven to a moderate temperature.
5. Pluck the rosemary leaves off their stems, leaving only the ends pieces in place.
6. Rub your salt and pepper from the kebab's ingredients into the lamb and eggplant cubes.
7. Drizzle the olive oil over the cubes now and toss them to have an even coat.
8. Sprinkle the lemon juice over the cubes and rub the rosemary stems between the cubes.
9. Skewer your lamb cubes by alternating each one with an eggplant cube.
10. Place the kebabs on an oven-proof dish in the center of the oven.
11. The kebabs will cook for 10 minutes, but you must turn them every 2 ½ minutes.
12. Take them out and let them rest for two minutes.
13. Enjoy the kebabs with the Salsa Verde.
14. Add a vegetable dish on the side for maximum nutrients.

Jaw-Dropping Ribeye (Lunch or Dinner)

This will be another choice to add a side vegetable dish to. Remember to use organic ribeye steak to avoid all the chemicals in the factory meat.

Serves: Two

Prep Time: 10 minutes
Cooking Time: 10 minutes
Ingredients:

- 1.2 lbs ribeye steak
- 2 tbsps olive oil
- 1 oz freshly-filleted anchovies
- 1 tbsp dried basil
- 1 clove crushed garlic
- 1 Pinch Himalayan salt and freshly-ground pepper
- 1 stick butter
- 1 tbsp freshly-squeezed lemon juice

Directions:

1. Finely chop the anchovy fillets and cream them into the butter.
2. Add the lemon juice and the salt and pepper.
3. Turn your grill onto moderate heat.
4. Rub the ribeye steak in the crushed garlic, coating every corner.
5. Season the steak with salt and pepper.
6. Mix the basil into the olive oil and coat your steak with it, too.
7. Drop the anchovy butter into the hot pan and let it melt.
8. Drop your steak in and grill it on one side for five minutes before turning it over.
9. You want the blood to start surfacing on the one side before flipping it, or it won't seal and be tender.

10. Reduce grill times to four or three minutes per side if you prefer rare steak.

Tangy Salmon (Lunch or Dinner)

I can't skip a fish recipe when it's packed with omega-3 and healthy nutrients. This dish will also still require a side dish of superfood vegetables.

Serves: Two
Prep Time: 10 minutes
Cooking Time: 10 minutes
Ingredients:

- 8 oz fresh salmon
- 3 tbsps butter
- 1 tbsp fresh lemon rind
- ¼ cup almond flour
- 1 tsp dill
- 1 tsp chives
- 1 tsp freshly-crushed garlic
- 2 tbsps finely-chopped spring onions
- A dash of sea salt and pepper

Directions:

1. Mix the almond flour, spring onions, garlic, dill, salt, and pepper on a large plate.
2. Press the salmon gently into the flour mixture and turn it over to coat both sides.
3. Do the same with the second salmon fillet.
4. Heat half of the butter and lemon zest in a skillet on medium heat until the butter melts.

5. Too much heat will burn the butter or make the rind bitter.
6. Drop the salmon in for three to four minutes on one side while you toggle the pan around to coat the fish well.
7. Wait for the butter to dry up and then turn the fish over.
8. Drop the remainder of the butter into the skillet and keep toggling it to coat the fish again.
9. Both sides should be crisp and you can use a fork to test the fish.
10. Remove the fish from the pan before it's fully cooked or it will overcook.
11. Let it rest for two minutes.

Roasted Superfood Side (Lunch or Dinner)

It's time to roast your side veggies by using the second-level superfoods that are best cooked to release nutrients and vitamins.

Serves: Four
Prep Time: 10 minutes
Cooking Time: 30 minutes
Ingredients:

- 1 cup cut broccoli
- 1 cup cut cauliflower
- 1 cup sliced zucchini
- 1 cup roughly chopped bell peppers (add some colors again)
- 1 cup roughly chopped onion
- 1 cup diced green beans

- ¼ cup of olive oil
- 2 tbsps balsamic vinegar
- 2 freshly-crushed garlic cloves
- 1 tsp sea salt
- ½ tsp freshly-ground pepper
- ½ tsp dried thyme
- ½ tsp dried oregano
- ½ tsp dried rosemary
- ½ tsp dried basil

Directions:

1. Preheat your oven to a hot temperature.
2. Line a baking tray with foil.
3. Throw all the onions, cauliflower, broccoli, zucchini, bell peppers, and green beans in a large bowl.
4. Whisk the olive oil, balsamic vinegar, salt, pepper, and herbs in a small bowl.
5. Pour the oily mixture over your vegetables and toss them to cover them all.
6. Place the vegetables in a single layer on the foil. You can use two baking pans if necessary, but you don't want the vegetables overcrowded.
7. Roast the veggies for 30 minutes and enjoy the golden-brown goodness of superfood sides.

Cauliflower Stir-Fry Side (Lunch or Dinner)

Cauliflower remains the most versatile vegetable that you can turn into anything; however, the internet is already full of rice, mash, and pizza recipes. Let's try something new.

Serves: Two
Prep Time: 15 minutes
Cooking Time: 15 minutes
Ingredients:

- ½ cup diced spring onions
- 1 small cauliflower head
- 2 large eggs
- ¼ cup chopped bell peppers
- 3 tbsps coconut oil
- 1 finely-diced piece of organic bacon
- 1/3 cup fresh peas (previously blanched or cooked)
- 3 tbsps wheat-free soy sauce
- 1 tsp peanut oil

Directions:

1. Whisk the eggs lightly and set it aside.
2. Grate the cauliflower and set it aside.
3. Scramble your eggs in a separate pan and set them aside.
4. Heat your wok on a high temperature.
5. Add the coconut oil and bacon to the wok.
6. Cook until the bacon is crisp. Be sure to stir the wok constantly as stir-fries burn easily.
7. Add your grated cauliflower and keep stirring.
8. Add the peanut oil and keep shaking the pan.
9. Throw your peas, spring onions, and bell peppers into the wok while stirring.
10. Drizzle the soy sauce into the wok and keep shaking it.

11. Add your scrambled eggs and stir like mad for two minutes.

12. Don't allow anything to burn because the flavors will swirl in your mouth if you get this right.

Snack Attack Two!

I have to sneak one more snack into my favorite recipes. It's not so much a recipe as it is an on-the-go idea you can use for pre-cooked chicken strips. You can decide what goes into the wraps, but this is my favorite version.

Serves: One
Prep Time: 10 minutes
Cooking Time: 5 minutes
Ingredients:

- 2 washed collard leaves
- ½ diced tomato
- ¼ cup organic cottage cheese
- 4 oz sliced chicken breast
- A dash of sea salt
- A dash of cayenne pepper (add more if you want because it's a great anti-inflammatory agent)
- 1 tbsp olive oil
- ¼ cup chopped cucumber

Directions:

1. Heat the pan at a moderate temperature and add your olive oil.
2. Season your chicken with salt and cayenne pepper.

3. Throw your sliced chicken breast in and give it a quick stir fry for no more than five minutes.
4. Lay the collard leaves flat on a plate and spread your cottage cheese over them.
5. Transfer the chicken from the pan to the collard leaves.
6. Sprinkle the tomatoes and cucumber over the chicken.
7. Wrap your collard leaves up like a burrito and enjoy!

Healthy Sweet Bombs!

How can I not throw in one of my favorite healthy treats? This is made of five ingredients and doesn't need to be unhealthy. Read your labels and eat this treat in moderation.

Makes: 12 Pieces (Six portions)
Prep Time: 10 minutes
Cooking Time: Zero!
Ingredients:

- 4 oz organic cream cheese
- 2 oz natural peanut butter
- 3 tbsps maple syrup
- ½ cup dark and organic chocolate chips
- 3 drops liquid Stevia

Directions:

1. Let the cream cheese and peanut butter reach room temperature first.

2. Combine the soft cheese, peanut butter, stevia, and maple syrup in a medium bowl.
3. Add the chocolate chips and blend them until the mixture is smooth.
4. Scoop small balls into your hand and line them in a flat, airtight container.
5. Freeze the balls for two hours to set them solid.

For more amazing recipes that follow the low-carb or complex carbohydrate idea, you can visit:
https://www.dietdoctor.com/low-carb/keto/recipes

Planning Your Meals

Planning your meals weekly seems like a complicated task, but it's quite simple if you know how to hone it. The fact that you have to buy more fresh produce because organic vegetables and fruits don't last as long, thus the reason why you must plan your meals weekly. You can purchase your ingredients every second week, but plan your meals by the week. The weekly planner below gives you an idea of the ingredients you're having throughout the week. Please note that the 'W' stands for an 8 oz glass of water. This means that you need to finish the number of glasses before the next meal. Study the plan before I explain it.

	W	Breakfast	W	Snack	W	Lunch	W	Snack	W	Dinner
Monday	1	eggs / fruit / bacon	2	fruit	2	snack board	2	chick wrap	1	beef / quinoa
Tuesday	1	steel-cut oats	2	yogurt	2	superfood veg salad	2	fruit	1	salmon / cauliflower
Wednesday	1	smoothie	2	nuts	2	quinoa salad	2	fruit	1	Monday night leftovers
Thursday	1	eggs / bacon / veg	2	fruit	2	snack board	2	carrot sticks	1	Tuesday night leftovers
Friday	1	smoothie	2	nuts	2	superfood salad / chicken	2	fruit	1	lamb / veggie roast
Saturday	1	steel-cut oats	2	fruit	2	Friday night leftovers	2	nuts	1	gluten-free pizza t/o
Sunday	1	omelette / veg / cheese	2	carrot sticks	2	salmon / superfoods veg	2	fruit	1	chicken wrap / superfoods

This seven-day planner makes eating clean simpler. You don't need to be precise about what you're eating with any given meal. State your meat or protein, what you'll add to it, and have a few flexible options. Otherwise, you'll overwhelm yourself. For example, snacks are optional, and you don't have to eat them, but you're giving yourself ideas ahead of time. Breakfasts are pretty straightforward. You can do anything with the eggs, bacon, and fruit. You can also make any recipe you find with the steel-cut oats. Smoothies have a myriad of options, and you can even experiment with different flavors. Try to have some superfoods in them as well.

Your lunch options are also flexible. You can pack anything on a snack board. I would add bits of chopped fruit, carrot sticks, cream cheese, cucumber, and even pieces of meat. The idea is to eat something of everything you put on the board. Snack boards are great for families because the kids can eat on the go. Add color and spunk to each snack board you make. The quinoa salad is also flexible because you can use different recipes. You can also prepare it beforehand, meaning that you could eat Monday's leftover quinoa on Wednesday afternoon. Leftovers are another way of simplifying the planner.

Why must you cook every night if you're busy? Eat Monday's leftovers on Wednesday and Tuesday's leftovers on Thursday. Saturday afternoon is when you eat Friday's leftovers. The idea with the leftovers is that you cook less and don't eat the same food with every meal, every day. If you're like me, you'll prefer to make your main meal on a Sunday afternoon instead of the evening. I have a lighter meal on a Sunday evening. Finally, you'll notice a takeout entry on the Saturday lunch spot. You're allowed to have a healthy takeout, such as gluten-free pizza. You can also swap your takeout or restaurant meal to Sunday afternoon next week.

This menu will make it easier for you to shop for organic and clean ingredients every two weeks. Some pointers with shopping every second week are:

1. Buy what is freshest and put it at the back of your fridge. Older products are in the front.
2. Be conscious about expiry or "best before" dates.
3. Blanch your vegetables after shopping so that you can freeze them.
4. Buy one ripe product and one that looks like it needs another month to ripen.

Another trick I use is to purchase something unusual every time I shop. This keeps the menu from going stale with the same superfoods all the time. Try new veggies and stock up on the dry products you need. You'll get free-range eggs that last a month, and you'll purchase enough quinoa to last four weeks too. It's the fresh produce you buy every second week. Keep an eye on those labels to make sure you're buying organic products. Meal planning is nothing to be scared of when you've got a flexible idea of what you need.

THE ART OF INTERMITTENT FASTING

Chapter 7

You've most likely heard of intermittent fasting, and you've wondered what all the rave is about. Fasting is a practice as old as ancient religions, but science has also latched onto the immense benefits of intermittently pausing your consumption and restarting it with new energy, focus, and fat-burning results. It's been perfected to help you bring back your health. If only you knew what it could do to your body sooner!

Starving Your Body Briefly Does What?

Before you misunderstand anything, know that intermittent fasting isn't a fad diet. It's a way to plan your meal timing. You're simply planning your periods of not eating or consuming calories and the periods where you return to food to consolidate your calories again. So, get all diet ideas out of your mind. Thomas DeLauer is a nutritional expert who encourages intermittent fasting because he understands the vast benefits to your body (DeLauer, 2018). The reason he advises his clients to do it is that you can burn huge amounts of fat while maintaining your muscles.

Your muscle tone and density will also increase. Another physical benefit is the improvement of your vascular system. This is the circulating system that gets blood and lymph to every part of your body. This enhances your physical health because every organ and gland is receiving the oxygen and nutrients that make them work at their best. The arteries flowing through your body are also the exit for the toxins that build up. So, your appearance doesn't only change for the better when you lose weight and pump up your muscles; it also improves because your skin and complexion aren't toxic anymore.

Even your nails and hair get the nutrients they need to look better. Intermittent fasting doesn't only tone you down; it also makes you look great on the outside. It also encourages the body to release adrenaline, norepinephrine, and epinephrine to protect the muscles and burn fat to convert it to energy. Therefore, you're burning fat for energy instead of relying on carbs. The mental benefits come when you're fasting and the brain switches over to survival mode. The survival mode is normally bad, but in short spurts, it can improve your focus because your alertness levels peak.

The survival mode will also require the brain to use the energy it has to sort through tasks. So, you won't be flooded with unwanted thoughts when you need to focus on one task. Your liver also starts producing ketones that target fat cells because there aren't any carbs left to convert to energy. Ketones are the fat-burning response that your brain triggers when it's losing carbohydrate energy. They're also called brain fuel because your neurons fire at higher rates when the energy comes from fat. Finally, intermittent fasting also regenerates your cells.

This meal timing plan triggers a process called autophagy, which is the regeneration of cells throughout your body. New and healthy cells will eat the old, diseased cells. This consolidates the new cells into more powerful cells. Cellular regeneration makes your skin glow, extends your life, and it improves the function of every organ in your body. If these benefits don't tempt you, then nothing will.

How to Start Your Intermittent Journey

Are your engines revving to know more? Well, there are some dos and don'ts to learn about before locking your food cabinet up for the day. Starting intermittent fasting sounds as simple as putting padlocks on every cabinet and the fridge, but there are some guidelines for before, during, and after your fast. You need to maintain your body correctly to avoid contradicting the fast. The fast period is what it's called when you go for a few hours without food, and the eating window is when you restore calories. The fast break is the first time you eat after fasting.

Do Prepare for the Fast

What you eat before fasting matters. Eat a high fiber meal before you start so that your body has some energy source to break down first. Let's say that you're fasting from 10:00 PM tonight until 2:00 PM tomorrow. Eat some high-fiber vegetables, such as broccoli, kale, collard greens, or Brussel sprouts at 10:00 PM to make sure your body can sustain the fast. You'll feel fuller for longer and won't wake up with a hungry grumble. Having some free fatty acids before your fast is also a good idea. Omega-3 fish, organic meat with some fat, and olive oil can be added to your late vegetable preparation. This will help your body produce ketones. Protein is also a necessity to maintain your body through the fast period.

Do Determine How Long You Want to Fast

The length of your fasting period will be dependent on the benefits you wish to achieve. Shorter fasts will produce some physical and mental benefits, but longer fasts will trigger the cellular regeneration effect. You could start with a 16-hour fast until you're ready for longer periods. This is called the 16-8 intermittent fast. It means that you must fast for 16 hours and eat calories for eight hours. Obviously, you're not eating for eight hours straight. The secret with this method is to make sure your eight hours are later in the day. Don't give yourself eight hours to eat away from morning to late afternoon.

Start your 16-hour fast at 10:00 PM so that you only have so many hours as an eating window. Start extending your fast times when you're ready, because 16 hours is the minimum of what's needed to activate the ketosis effect. After this, you can start adding an hour to every fast period until you're comfortable. Every hour you add will come with multiplied benefits. People who use prolonged fasts that last between 24 and 48 hours reach a new state of mental sharpness. The body composition benefits don't multiply anymore, but the mental benefits and cellular regeneration keep snowballing.

Do Know What You Can Consume During Your Fast

You're allowed to drink black coffee without sweetener or creamer. Black coffee can actually speed up the autophagy in your body to regenerate new cells. Cell Cycle Journal published an interesting article (Pietrocola et al., 2014). They induced autophagy in the heart, liver, and muscles with caffeinated and decaffeinated black coffee in mice.

The second benefit was established when the polyphenols in coffee reduced active proteins that slowed the metabolism down. Both results proved that black coffee is a great fasting supplement. You can also drink black or green tea without sweetener or creamer. Purified water is another safe drink that you can have as much of as you wish. The only time you won't drink water or black coffee is when you're on a dry fast.

Don't Consume the Wrong Stuff

Bullet-proof coffee makes the rounds on the internet for dietary reasons. It requires you to add butter or some form of healthy fat to your coffee, but it doesn't work for intermittent fasting. Calories shouldn't be consumed during your fast period, whether it's from food, snacks, or drinks. Stay away from diet sodas, too, because the artificial sweetener will trigger your insulin levels and stop the autophagy. Insulin spikes will trigger a metabolic response that messes your fast up.

Consider your fast broken if this happens. Broth is another common mistake people make during a fast. You're still consuming calories, even with bone broth. Alcohol is another fast-breaker. Your body converts alcohol into acetaldehyde, which is also known as a carcinogen. Because acetaldehyde is so toxic, the metabolism will prioritize it. The liver needs to process the toxin, and it can't release the ketones needed to burn fat. Alcohol should only be consumed if necessary, a few hours after you break your fast with food.

Don't Take Pre-Workout Supplements

Pre-workout meals, smoothies, and protein shakes can also break your fast. Branched-chain amino acid supplements (BCAAs) should be avoided during a fast. They include leucine, valine, and isoleucine that promote higher proteins in the body that will only offset the cellular regeneration, breaking your fast. You're using a physiological and natural process to maintain muscle mass, and you don't need the supplements during this period.

Don't Use the Wrong Nutrient Supplements

Do your supplements contain carbs or calories? If so, they'll break your fast. Any supplements in a soft gel coat will also break a fast, such as fish oil supplements. You can take your water-soluble multivitamins during your fast. Try to take them during your eating window even though they don't break your fast, because they'll be tough on the stomach when it's empty.

Do Break Your Fast With Bone Broth

I'm sure you know that eating three hamburgers and two slabs of chocolate isn't the way to break your fast, but some people do it wrong anyway. Having a life-long health goal means that you must always respect your body. Breaking a fast with a bone broth is a great option. Cook bones in hot water with some natural flavors and some vegetables because this activates the collagen proteins to keep the gut healthy. Your gut mucosal layer temporarily weakens during a fast, and that's why you need to restore it. The mucosal layer is the gut lining that prevents damage from acids. Eating four to six ounces of bone broth will help the stomach lining absorb the nutrients and prevent damage from other foods.

Don't Break Your Fast With Carbs and Fats Combined

Combining carbs and fats right after a fast is bad. The carbs will immediately spike your insulin, and your cells will be highly receptive to what you're eating right after the fast. Therefore, combining carbs and fats will allow your cells to absorb insulin, which makes the cells open to collecting what you eat. Consuming carbs alone after a fast will encourage the cells to absorb the carbs, but consuming fat alone means that the cells won't absorb it because there's no insulin spike. Rather, have carbs and protein together, or eat fats and protein together when breaking your fast.

Do Workout During the Fast

You could workout during your fast or after you break it, but working out can speed up the ketosis process to burn fat and preserve muscle mass. The lipid fats stored in your muscles will be expelled into the bloodstream to be converted into energy when you work out while your body is already in the fasting stage. The Journal of Physiology published the results from studies conducted on fasting versus skipped breakfast participants (Edinburgh et al., 2018). Fasting men were burning more fat than those who simply skipped breakfast when they were working out before the break of their fast.

If you start your fast at 10:00 PM, workout in the morning, and eat at 2:00 PM again, then you've had a few hours of heightened ketosis. However, working out just before you break your fast is also an option. Your body is already tired, and it's busy burning fat before you push it to burn more. The problem with the second option is that you'll struggle to perform because your body is tired. If you want to workout after you break the fast, make sure you're giving your body a chance to digest the food first. All your blood will be flowing to the organs to help the digestion process, so exercising will encourage the blood to move away from the organs, and you'll miss out on key nutrients.

Don't Confuse Intermittent Fasting With Liquid Fasting

Liquid fasting allows you to still consume bullet-proof coffee, broths, and other liquid meals. You're still consuming calories which only spike your insulin. Liquid fasts don't offer the metabolic benefits of intermittent fasting; they simply give your body a break from solid foods.

Don't Confuse Intermittent Fasting With Dry Fasting

Dry fasting is an extreme method people use sparingly. It removes all liquids and not just food. It even removes water from your fast period. Dry fasting uses a different system. It encourages your body to pull hydrogen from your fat cells to convert it to water. It's an extreme method used for weight loss because the body is forced to burn fat to make water.

Do Know That Men and Women Differ Slightly

Men and women's metabolisms work similarly, except for one difference. Women have a complex reproductive system that sends more intense hunger signals during a fast. Their survival mode from the brain is always considering the reproductive organs, even if there isn't a baby to nourish. Women may want to start with shorter fasts of 12 hours and then work their way up from that.

Common Concerns

Fasting has a few misconceptions attached. The first one is that people believe they're going to lose muscle mass. The Journal of Translational Medicine published a study conducted on 34 men divided into two groups (Moro et al., 2016). The first group of resistance-trained men were placed on a 16-8-hour intermittent fasting plan for eight weeks, and the other group were partaking in a regular diet with the same calories for the same period. Both groups were tested before and after the program to establish muscle mass, fat mass, and health biomarkers that determine the risk they had of heart disease.

Firstly, the intermittent fasting group showed more muscle gain after the eight weeks than the regular guys. They also showed significantly less fat mass and their biomarkers improved. Another concern is the thyroid because people think it will slow down. Thyroids slow down when we consume fewer calories, but intermittent fasting gives us a window to eat our calories daily. So, there's no chance of permanently slowing down your metabolism or thyroid function. Logically, your thyroid slows down during the fast period, but it starts producing hormones as soon as you eat again.

Planning Your Fast

Your intermittent fasting will need to apply all the dos and don'ts you learned about. I've created a simple chart to help you design a seven-day 16-8-hour fast. Feel free to customize it to suit your needs better. You can also fast intermittently for seven days and take a break, or you can go for two weeks. Don't exceed two weeks at a time. Rather fast intermittently for two weeks every second month.

	Monday	Tuesday	Wednesday	Thursday	Friday	Saturday	Sunday
8:00 AM	workout/water	workout/water	water	workout/water	workout/water	workout/water	black coffee
9:00 AM	water	tea	tea	water	tea	water	water
10:00 AM	tea	water	water	black coffee	water	water	tea
11:00 AM	water	black coffee	water	water	black coffee	tea	water
12:00 PM	black coffee	water	water	black coffee	tea	water	black coffee
1:00 PM	water	tea	tea	water	water	black coffee	water
2:00 PM	bone broth	vegetable broth	fat/no carbs	light carbs/no fat	superfood broth	fat/no carbs	superfood carbs
3:00 PM	water	tea	water	tea	water	tea	water
4:00 PM	lunch	lunch	lunch	lunch	lunch	lunch	lunch
5:00 PM	tea	water	black coffee	water	tea	water	black coffee
6:00 PM	dinner	dinner	dinner	dinner	dinner	dinner	dinner
7:00 PM	black coffee	water	water	tea	water	water	tea
8:00 PM	water	water	tea	water	water	black coffee	water
9:00 PM	snack	snack	black coffee	snack	snack	water	snack
10:00 PM	protein/fiber/fat	protein/fiber/fat	protein/fiber/fat	protein/fiber/fat	protein/fiber/fat	protein/fiber/fat	protein/fiber/fat

Now, you have one more method of correcting your health. Use intermittent fasting at least three times a year to restore the cells in your body.

YOU CAN'T JUST SIT AROUND

Chapter 8

All the evidence points to being active to be healthy. The only time you don't train is during a detox, but clean eating and intermittent fasting are complemented by workouts. Unfortunately, we don't all have the time or money to spend hours at the gym. Bring the gym to your home at times like these. You'll learn about some great exercises and the minimal equipment you need to keep at home to turn your spare room into a home gym. There's something for everyone, from strenuous muscle-building exercises to literal walks in the park.

Resistance Band Training

Resistance bands are affordable home gym equipment that comes with many benefits. The first is obvious because the more you pull on the elastic band, the more it resists, creating a good workout for muscle tone and mass. It's an improvement to dumbbells because some positions, such as the biceps curl, become easier when you near the top twist with a dumbbell. Resistance bands become harder, straining your muscles further. You have to tense your muscles even harder to fight the resistance from the band, making sure your muscles groups get the workout they need if you plan to tone your body or build more muscle mass.

Resistance bands take up no space in your home gym, and they don't break the bank. They can be used to complement other equipment. You can use one standard band loop to create challenging workouts in every area of your home that promotes bodybuilding enhancements. You can even use it during your squats or push-ups to add some resistance. Loop your band around your bedposts, banisters, or pillars to turn your home into a rowing gym. Hook it onto a tree branch and work your triceps on a pulldown. The options are endless. Let's look at a few simple options.

One: Work Those Arms

Position yourself for a single-arm reverse fly by standing upright, wrapping your band around the back of your left shoulder, and bringing it around the right bicep so that you can tug it with your left hand. Hold your arms in front of you while the loop is attached to the left, and swing them backward like you're flying. You'll feel a lot of resistance on your left arm. Continue flapping for 30 counts, and switch the loop to the opposite shoulder.

Two: Tone the Butt

Position yourself for a forward-scissored squat. Your left knee is touching the ground, and your right foot is flat with the knee bent at 90 degrees. Strap the band under your right foot, and raise your right hand to be flush with your face while it holds the other end of the loop. Position your left arm straight against your side. Now, rise and drop like you're squatting. Do this for another 30 counts and switch legs.

Three: Work Your Biceps

Stand with your knees slightly bent after putting your band under your feet. Hold the other end of the band in both hands, and bend over to create a short tension between the foot and hand loops. Now, straighten your back as you pull tight on the band and bend over again. Do this for 30 counts. It should look like you're rowing in an upright position.

Four: Work Your Abs and Triceps

Lay on your back, and run both sides of the loops around your feet without putting pressure on your ankles. Always make sure the loops are gentle on the ankles. Bend your knees, and grab the center of the loop to rest it above your pelvis. Raise your butt as high as you can to form a bridge shape. Your elbows are supporting you. Drop the bridge, and do it for another 30 counts.

Five: Full Body Workout

Sit with your legs flat against the floor, and hook one end of the loop under your feet. Hold the other end in both hands and start rowing back and forth by lowering your back and raising it. Always keep your spine as straight as possible while doing this.

There are countless ideas with resistance bands. These are five easy techniques you can try.

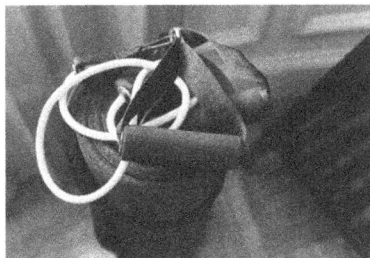

Resistance Bands

Walking

Walking should never be underrated as a workout. It's an aerobic exercise that gets your blood flowing and your heart pumping healthily. Aerobic exercises come with many health benefits you won't want to dismiss (Frey & Stanten, 2020). It improves heart health in people who lead both healthy and chronic lives. Your risk of heart failure caused by menopause is also reduced by 25%. It's understandable if you're doing a cardiovascular routine because better blood flow makes sure that every organ receives the required nutrients and oxygen.

High-density lipoprotein (HDL) is also enhanced with aerobic exercise. HDL is the good kind of cholesterol you need in your body. Non-HDL is the bad kind. Low-density lipoprotein (LDL) cholesterol is also associated with heart disease. Good cholesterol has antioxidant and anti-inflammatory properties to help the immune system stay strong. Your blood pressure is lowered, and your risk for type two diabetes is decreased by 50%. Depending on the routine you have, you could be dropping calories, too. The brain also releases feel-good chemicals when you're walking through the park, and this counters stress and negative emotions, leading to better mental health.

Adding some weight-bearing exercises to your walking routine also counteracts the gravitational forces that make people's bones degenerate, leaving you with a lower risk of osteoporosis and arthritis. Overall, combining aerobic exercises with healthy lifestyles will prolong your longevity because it counters the risk of so many diseases. However, you can't simply spend 10 minutes walking daily if you're not adding additional training. Aim for 30 minutes daily if you walk five days a week, or 21 minutes daily if you walk every day. This will get your heart pumping the way it should.

Add nature to your walks, too, because this can further benefit you mentally. So, walk through parks if you must, but keep at it for the minimally-required times. Finally, don't stroll casually. Treat it as an exercise by walking briskly or power-walking.

Cycling

Cycling also comes with a myriad of health benefits (Minnis & Cronkleton, 2020). You can manage your weight, build muscle strength in your legs, and it targets the core muscles and back. Your mental health is boosted when feel-good chemicals are transmitted again, and your stress will be managed properly, keeping cortisol balanced. Cycling also works to create better blood flow, reducing blood pressure, bad cholesterol, and improving heart health. It lowers the risk of type two diabetes and lessens the chance of having a stroke. It's a low-impact exercise routine that doesn't put additional pressure on the joints.

Your balance, posture, and coordination will also improve because cycling requires all three to fight the effects of gravity. Keeping your weight under control also reduces the risk of certain cancers, such as breast cancer. In fact, cancer patients are often advised to cycle to keep their symptoms under control. It counteracts the fatigue brought on by chemotherapy. It's a great option for beginners and doesn't require anything but a bicycle. Adding nature also doesn't hurt, but you need to be conscious about your routes for safety.

Always consider safety when cycling. Use the lanes provided, and never think you won't fall. Buy a helmet and reflective clothing to make you visible in the bike lane. Also, never cycle through existing pain or tension in the muscles. You might have an injury and worsen it. Use the lowest intensity gear on your bicycle, and cycle for 30 minutes daily. Take one day weekly as a break, because it's a full workout on your body.

Push-Ups

This is an age-old classic that requires no equipment but rather determination, motivation, and discipline. It's a strength and muscle-building workout used by top athletes globally. What most people don't realize is that there are numerous right ways of doing push-ups.

Method One: Planking

Planking was inspired by push-ups and didn't fall from the sky. The most effective push-ups start with a rigid plank position. Press your elbows against the ground, and close your hands together to make a triangle. Dig your toes into the ground to give yourself a lift on the balls of your feet. Your back, shoulders, neck, butt, and calves must run in a solid line. Your spine must always be straight, and your head should face the triangle to reduce unwanted strain on your neck muscles. Stay in this position for 60 seconds. You might start with 30 seconds and work your way toward bigger goals. Planking is a full-body workout that could be done three times daily if you have the energy for it. Otherwise, work your way toward three times.

Method Two: Wise Hands

This push-up works on your core and upper-body muscles. This is the position most people are familiar with when doing push-ups. Lay flat on your stomach with your chin touching the ground. Curl your toes inward to support the lift on the balls of your feet. Place your hands palm-down just below your chin. Your fingers should be close to touching each other. Now, keep your back and legs straight while you push yourself away with your hands and support yourself with your feet balls. Do 20 push-ups in this position when you start and increase them with five every week.

Method Three: Hindu Push

This push-up will work on your core muscles, triceps, and shoulders while improving your flexibility. You're going to go into a downward dog yoga position by bending your body into a triangle shape while resting your upper body on your hands and your lower body on the balls of your feet. Inch yourself forward until your chin touches the floor. Then, use your arms to push your upper body forward and raise it into the cobra position. Now, your legs will be against the floor, and your head will be pointing to the ceiling. Maintain this position for 60 seconds at a time, and release it in the reverse method of how you entered it, being careful not to pull a muscle.

Method Four: Sidekick Push-Up

Adding a sideways kick to a traditional push-up works wonders for the core muscles. Lay on the floor with your elbows raised and your chin on the ground. Use the balls of your feet to support yourself as your hands push you up. Now, this requires balance, but you'll have to lower your chin slightly and bring one leg closer to your butt. Slowly move it along your supported calf, and then you can extend it. Don't be abrupt with this, because you can hurt your muscles. Bring it back in, and slowly move it down your calf again. Repeat this five times and switch to the other leg.

Push-ups aren't as boring as the gym teacher made you think. There are countless methods available. Look for more on YouTube.

Squats

Squats are known for toning your butt and making it look like the perfect curve on your body. They also work on your triceps, legs, and core muscles. And guess what? There are multiple methods to squat as well, and I don't mean the type where you squat in someone's home.

Squat One: Traditional

Stand with a straight posture, and shift your shoulders back a hint. Spread your feet as wide as your shoulders with your feet pointing forward. Now, drop your butt toward the floor without making your knees cave. Let your knees support the drop, and don't bend your spine too much. Move your hands forward as you drop. You want to straighten your arms in front of you. Your shoulders will move forward, but you must focus on balance and keeping your spine straight. Stay down for the count of three and spring back up. Continue doing this another 20 counts.

Squat Two: Goblet Squat

This squat works on the butt, core muscles, and upper-body. You'll need a dumbbell or anything with two or three pounds of weight. Please note that you can add your resistance band to this exercise, too. Stand in the same position you were in with the traditional squat, except your legs are only hip-width apart this time. Hold your dumbbell in the center of your chest with both hands, and bend your knees for a gentle, balanced drop. Be kinder to your shoulders now as the weight will also pull them forward more this time. Continue dropping and rising for 20 counts.

Squat Three: Ball Squat

This one is more complicated, but it gives you a fuller workout. It targets the core muscles, back, shoulders, legs, triceps, and biceps to make a near-perfect all-rounder. You'll need a ball for this squat. Try using a heavier ball as this squat is best with a heavy medicine ball that weighs you down. You can also use a two or three-pound dumbbell if you want to. Otherwise, use a small rock from the garden. You're going to start by standing on one leg. The ball is in front of you and will extend as your arms straighten when you drop. Your knee from the standing leg will bend when you drop, and the other leg will extend forward. Bring the extended leg back when you rise and rest it on your standing calf. Do 15 drops like this, and then you can alternate to the other leg.

Squat Four: Jumping Squats

Jumping squats also target the butt, core muscles, and triceps. The jump will offer some benefits for the gravitational force you're fighting. Enter the traditional squat pose and drop down. Think of this exercise as the jumping jack of squats. So, you're going to jump when you rise. Try to keep your balance as you aim for 20 of these squats.

Experiment with your squats, and see what you can

come up with. Just remember that exercise shouldn't cause intense pain. That would mean that you're positioning yourself wrong.

Foam Roll Stretching

Stretching your muscles has vast benefits of its own (Yeun & Bubnis, 2018). It alleviates pain and reduces muscle inflammation. It also helps the muscles repair themselves without too much strain. Stretching your muscles also makes them more flexible, and you'll be less likely to injure them in the future. Your blood flow improves when you reduce the inflammation and you find better relaxation. The problem is that not everyone has time or funds to join a yoga class. That's where foam rolls come in handy. You won't believe what muscle groups you can target with a piece of silly foam that costs virtually nothing.

Foam Roll One: Quads

Your quad muscles at the top of your legs probably need some exercise if you've been sedentary. It's easy to work on them with the foam roller. Place yourself in a simple plank position with the noodle under your quads. Keep your upper body supported on your elbows and arms as you start rolling back and forth. Allow the foam roller to roll under your core muscles down to the quads. Hold your position for 20 seconds if you find a tender spot. Continue doing this for 30 to 60 seconds.

Foam Roll Two: Hip Rolling

This one works for inflamed and painful hips. You'll be flexing the muscles in your hips and the tissues surrounding them. Find yourself in the same position as the quad roll, and support your upper body on your forearms that lie flat against the floor. Bend your right leg comfortably to your side, and rest your left hip on the roller. Start rolling back and forth, and from side to side, noticing any tender spots. Tender spots always require 20 minutes of pressure before moving on. Roll this hip for 30 to 60 seconds and switch to the other side.

Foam Roll Three: Roll Those Calves

This roll relaxes the calf muscles and is loads of fun anyway. Sit on the floor, and place the roller under your calves. Rest your body backward by placing your arms and hands slightly behind your hips. Raise your butt from the floor and roll back and forth as though you're rocking.

Foam Roll Four: Rolling the Back

Everyone gets back pain from time to time, so it's a good idea to have a stretch for it. Ladies, make sure your hair is out of the way otherwise you won't enjoy this one! Lay on your back and bend your knees. Place both arms in a hug position over your chest once you've placed the noodle under your back. Use your legs to raise your back gently, and start rolling back and forth. Focus on the upper-back for now. You can do the lower-back with the next repetition. Move gently and don't strain yourself. Look for the tender spots and press on them.

Exercise and being active is a huge part of being healthy. Depending on what your long-term goals are, you can choose between aerobic, gentle, brisk, or strenuous exercises. Just promise yourself that you'll start.

HEALING THE MIND, BODY, AND SOUL

Chapter 9

The final piece of your longer, healthier, and happier lifestyle is to focus on the mind, body, and soul connection. You've learned about the science that links the gut and brain, how the brain is the master puppeteer, and how it's influenced by the gut. Now, it's time to learn how to heal your mental and emotional state naturally. Holistic methods can target the alternative connection between the mind and body to give you clarity and relief. Your journey isn't complete without healing every part of yourself.

Energy Healing

Science might call it particles, but alternative healers call the life-force inside of you 'energy.' There are similarities between modern medicine and holistic practices. Science links the gut, immune system, endocrine system, and CNS into one harmonious flow of particles. Energy healers connect the body through chakras. You have seven major chakras that interconnect, but there's a total of 114 chakras throughout the body. Energy healers or Reiki practitioners have opened their hand chakras to allow energy manipulation and replacement. They use their hands to guide, balance, heal, or restore your energy that lacks in certain regions. Understand what your seven major chakras or energy centers are before undertaking energy healing.

You have the root chakra starting at your tailbone, which is the point of your body that connects to the earth. The grounding chakra is where our senses of belonging and survival come from. You'll feel financially or emotionally insecure if this chakra is misaligned. Fear or anxiety also indicates that it's unbalanced.

Then you have the sacral chakra that lies in your pelvic region under the navel. This chakra is important because it's where your motivation lies to seek the true pleasure of life, including intimacy, good and clean nutrition, and abundance without seeking more than you can handle. Addiction, gluttony, obesity, and hormonal imbalances are often tied to this energy center if it's unbalanced.

The solar plexus or core chakra is the center of your stomach. It connects to your gut and is responsible for your confidence, identity, wisdom, and inner-strength. An overactive core chakra causes digestive issues. It can also lead to problems with the kidneys, pancreas, and liver. You might feel insecure and emotionally dependent on others if it's blocked.

The heart chakra is where your love, compassion, and kindness come from, including self-love and self-compassion. Unbalanced heart chakras cause poor relationships, palpitations, and circulation problems. You might also feel guarded and unloved if you don't restore the energy.

The throat chakra signifies your inner truth, purity, and clarity. You'll be able to speak honestly when you open it. Frequent throat infections and digestive issues show an imbalance. Emotionally, you'll fear speaking the truth that ties to the source of your happiness.

The third-eye chakra is behind your forehead, representing the mind. It's the gateway into the mind itself and is commonly opened through energy healing and meditation. It connects to the five senses and allows you to feel balanced in life. It's where intuition and self-development lie. Migraines are a physical symptom of imbalance, but you'll be feeling detached from the world emotionally.

The crown chakra is the final major energy center, and it's on top of your head, also connecting to your mind. This is where your consciousness, health, happiness, wisdom, spirituality, and purpose reside. Every decision you make is made best through a higher purpose, including health decisions. Your mind will be swamped with unwanted thoughts if this one is blocked.

Now, you can focus on opening the stream that flows from the crown chakra to the root chakra, or vice versa by visiting an energy healer. You can learn to heal these pathways yourself, but it helps to start with a healer. You must watch them and allow them to guide you. Some energy healers will even use their eyes or voice to heal your centers. Try to find one that uses their hands. You'll be practicing energy healing yourself in no time after a few visits to your Reiki practitioner. The main reason for mindfully witnessing an energy healer two or three times before conducting your own healing is that intentions play a big role.

Your intention guides your energy manipulation from your hands. When visiting a healer, you must state your intentions so that they know what's needed. Speak to them about the symptoms you're experiencing emotionally or physically, and allow them to guide you. They'll open the chakras once they set the intention for certain problems. For example, a blocked sacral chakra could be tied to an emotional battle with a clean, healthy lifestyle. Perhaps, you have IBS, and this could mean that your core chakra is blocked. One blocked chakra leads to others suffering because they run in a stream. It's also okay if you're unwilling to share your intentions at first.

However, in this case, you must go into the healing session with your intention clear in your mind. The healer's hands will either enter your energy field, touch you, or move gently over it in various techniques. Take notes so that you can perform

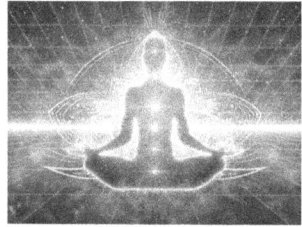

Chakra Stream

the same healing frequently once you've witnessed it mind-fully. Be open-minded because this will help the source of blocked energy to expose itself. Your healer will either pull bad energy out or they'll redirect it to recreate the flow that needs to run from your mind to your root. Here are some methods to use for energy healing, whether through a healer or your own hands.

The Field Scan

The healer will pass their hands over your energy field, within a few inches, assessing the current state of your energy centers. You'll lay on your back, and their down-ward palms will pass slowly from your feet to your head. You also need to be aware, alert, and open to the scan to feel the shifts of energy as their hands glide over it. The healer will feel changes in their hands if the energy is wrong, and you might feel sensations in the passing regions, too. The healers passing hands, or yours, will feel tingly, warm, cold, attracted, or repelled by problematic areas. Healers will get intuitive information from the scan, but you might feel epiphanies as they comb over your field too. The field scan is merely an assessment. There's no need to intentionally change the energy or diagnose the problems yet.

Still Hands Healing

This is the most common form of healing once imbalances are found. Your healer will place their still hands over the region to regulate the energy. Energy disturbances require hands in the field or touching the body, either still or moving slowly. You, the healer, or both, need to focus your intention on restoring the balance and flow in this region. The healer will follow their wise intuition about the center and only focus as long as they need to. Sometimes, the center's disturbance is part of a larger healing process. Other than the healer's energy regulating yours through their embrace, you can also use still hands healing at home. Our instincts tell us to touch a wounded area, and sometimes, this touch with the right intention is all that's needed.

Smooth Healing

A healer might also use sweeping motions to clear a field of disturbed energy. The motion of their hands will smooth the turmoil in the center, much like a massage or tickle makes a tender spot feel relaxed. The intention with smooth healing is to restore the energy to its natural state. Healers will continue a sweeping motion about six inches above your skin, starting from the disturbed area and moving outwards. Some healers sweep the entire energy field first, then return to the imbalanced area before sweeping from head to toes again.

Energy Pump Healing

This is a good option for pains, such as headaches and wounds. The healer holds their predominant hand over your painful region and extends their other hand to the ground. Their intention is set to pull the disrupted energy through the hand above you and send it into the ground through their other hand. They're taking your unwanted or painful energy into their bodies, and they'll need to pump their ground-facing fist quickly a few times before your pain diminishes totally, or they'll have built-up energy from you.

Magnetic Healing

The final option the healer uses is to hover their hands over your disturbed energy source, which can be caused by pain, trauma, emotional disturbances, or disease. They intend to magnetically pull the energy out of your field through their palms that are either touching you or hovering six inches over your skin. The healer uses their third-eye chakra to visualize the energy flooding out of your body, and it helps if you can do this, too. They imagine the energy sticking to their hands like glue, and so must you. They'll flick their hands toward the ground to shake off the energy they collect throughout the session.

Energy healing is a draining process, and you'll need to take a brisk walk outdoors when you're done. You can also ground yourself away from the disrupted energy by confirming yourself in front of a mirror. Tell the reflection what you do for a living, who you are, and what just happened. Energy healing isn't for everyone, but it does wonders when you set the right intentions and practice it enough to heal yourself.

Enter the Zen Mindspace

Zen meditation is another lifestyle you must adopt to be mindfully healthy. It's an ancient mindful practice from the Tang Dynasty around seventh-century China, and it can reduce stress, anxiety, blood pressure, and chronic symptoms (Mindworks Team, 2018). Added benefits are improved immune system functions, focus, and sleep. The word 'zen' translates to *ch'an*, which means insight into the workings of the mind. Learning the mind's frame inside and outside is how you cope with stress and unwanted thoughts or feelings. Entering the mind in a calm state brings you back to the present moment where you need to ground yourself to cope with stress.

You can't cope with it if your mind is stuck in tomorrow or yesterday. Happiness and a stress-free life only exist right here and now. It also goes much deeper than stress reduction. Zen meditation allows you to open your third-eye chakra, enhancing your focus and intuition. You can scan the mind and body to find deep-rooted issues that hold your perfect health back. You might also find answers to questions you've always had. It's the deepest form of introspection, and anyone can practice it. Practicing it enough can help you connect with the refined purpose inside of you as well.

Buddhists used zen meditation alongside transcendental meditation to reach spiritual highs and become one with Buddha himself. There's nothing wrong with knowing that there's a higher purpose or universal presence. It humbles us and opens our minds to caring for others, being a role model for kids, and being empathetic. Digging deeper into your mind is where you find the core issues you're struggling with in life. It can also help you see other people's core problems if you intend to help others. Being kind, considerate, and compassionate to other people is a classic zen tradition.

It enhances your well-being by sharing your positive energy with others. What you give the world will always come back to you, even if it's only in personal satisfaction. The truth is that everything is interconnected in the world. Your energy is interconnected with another person, and theirs is connected to someone else. Our chance for happiness and abundant health lies within us. Think of it as karma. The more happiness you share, the more emotional wealth you'll gain. Zen meditation teaches you to train your mind into a calmness where it can reflect, focus, be creative, and experience fulfillment.

Honing the meditation can lead to living a zazen lifestyle. Zazen is a particular form of meditation where you can enter a mindspace clear enough to understand the nature of existence. Knowing why we exist is how we ultimately heal our minds from anything that taints the mind, body, and soul connection. Observation, relaxation, introspection, mindfulness, and living in the present moment can be achieved through guided zen meditations on Headspace or YouTube. There are also simple methods to practice at home that offer fewer distractions.

Meditation requires practice, though, and you can start with guided sessions if you need to. Otherwise, practice any of the following zen techniques. For someone learning to meditate in zazen, it's advised to position yourself in the easy yoga pose until you learn to find your own comfort. Sit on a soft cushion, cross your legs comfortably, and rest your hands gently on your knees. Face your palms toward the sky like Buddhist monks do. Straighten your spine and shut your eyes. Now, you can use any of the methods.

Observation of Breath

Your posture is key during the observation of your breath, so the easy yoga pose works perfectly. You need to observe your breath flowing into your body and out of your mouth. Don't try to control your breath, but only follow it slowly as it pulls deep into your core muscles. Your stomach and entire diaphragm must fill every time you breathe in. Observe the sensations of the breath in your core, and follow it as it flows in and out, pushing it out entirely every time. Feel your belly rise and fall as your alertness and focus on the breath is the only thing on your mind. Continue following the flow for 10 minutes without interrupting it. Just feel the tickling sensation against your inner passageways.

Thoughtful Awareness

You're not going to focus on your breath in thoughtful awareness. You're going to shut your eyes and just be. Your mind is just as it is, and your thoughts flow through it freely without judgment. Sit in your comfortable position, and allow the thoughts to come to you. Let them pass through your mind because they're only thoughts. They have no physical weight, and they don't define you. You can't grasp or reject them. You can only watch them pass through like a slow-moving train traveling through the mind's station. Allow your mind to be what it is, and allow yourself to be who you are. Zazen doesn't provide a means to an end, it's the end itself. Just let these thoughts flow and dissipate on their own. You can remain in this state for 10 to 20 minutes daily.

Mindful Walk

Practicing a mindful walk takes time, but it's a great

reliever of stress and unwanted thoughts or emotions. Take a zen nature walk when you feel overwhelmed. Take it slow and steady as you absorb the environment through your senses. Listen to the birds in the trees, and smell the salt in the air if you're near the ocean. Kick your shoes off, and feel the ground beneath your toes. Look at the colors, shapes, and beauty of everything in nature. Welcome the sensory stimulants as you consume every sight, smell, sound, sensation, and taste on your walk. Just be you as you traipse through the park. You can also use mindful awareness during daily tasks. Cook a superfood roast, and engulf your senses in every step.

Intentional Change

Find yourself comfortable again, and simply scan your body and mind. What do you feel? Where do you feel it? How big is the sensation? Give all feelings and tenders spots in your body or mind a physical location and shape. Scan every inch of your body and accept what you find. Don't judge your findings, rather change your intentions toward them. Can you feel a heaviness over your heart? Is there a thought that stirs troubling emotions in your mind? You can't change it in your zen state. You can only set your intentions to change it in your life. This is another great method to use daily when you feel unwell mentally, emotionally, or physically. It teaches you to set intentions because you can't change what you don't intend to change.

Positive Contemplation

Shut your eyes in your easy yoga pose, and just be comfortable with yourself again. There's no need to focus intently on anything. Simply be, and allow the mind to be. Repeat your thoughtful awareness meditation, except this time you're going to contemplate different scenarios. Use your imagination to paint pictures in your mind. It might take a few minutes of being aware before you can paint pictures. Once you can, start designing thoughts you'd like to see on your mental train. Picture yourself healthy, happy, and prosperous. Use your senses inside your mind to piece together a perfect image of who you want to be. How do you want to look, sound, and smell? Where are you and what do you see around you? Keep painting images in your mind after completing your thoughtful awareness sessions. These images align with your desires, dreams, and goals.

Leading a zen life is simple. Energy healing is simple. However, the two combined can offer you an outlet for anything standing between you and the consolidation of your mind, body, and soul. Once consolidated, your emotions, symptoms, and stresses will stop flowing into your body.

AFTERWORD

Being healthy and living a well-deserved life hasn't been this close to your grasp before. I suspect that you're tired of leading the life you once did. Who wouldn't be sick of being exhausted and dragging their feet all day long? You can't keep living with the pains, bloatedness, inflammation, and unexplained headaches for the rest of your life.

No one could be happy with the digestive problems that lead to some embarrassing moments. You don't need to wake up to breakfast with a side of 50 medications anymore. Even young people know this terrible curse. The doctors keep giving you more, and all you want to do is flush them down the toilet.

Being sick isn't the life anyone wants, whether it's chronic, serious, severe, mild, or simply irritating. Often, the medicine prescribed only makes you feel worse. What about the food you're exposed to? You think you're living healthily, following fad diet after fad diet, but you're still showing those inescapable love handles. Your stomach won't flatten, and you're sure you have diabetes.

Poor nutrition and ill-health go hand-in-hand. The funny fact is that we drown our depression in food as well, even though some foods cause it. Chronic conditions can lead to more complications, and modern, pasteurized, preserved, chemicalized food doesn't make it any better. Instead, we find ourselves back at the doctor's office, filling a new prescription.

It's a vicious cycle that seems never-ending. We become sedentary when our bodies feel like they've been minced inside, leading to more trouble. The cycle turns into an avalanche of poor health and unhappy lives. Health and happiness are also intertwined. We must never forget that we can't be happy when we're sick all the time. We can't be happy when we feel depressed, eat poorly, or abstain from exercise.

How can we be happy when our minds and bodies work against us? Fortunately, you've learned how to combat this now. You know the biological processes inside the body and how each system affects another one. You know how the food industry uses products that shouldn't be allowed on animals. The cover-ups can't hide anymore with all the evidence readily available on the internet.

You just needed someone to put it together neatly so that you can apply the practical methods of correcting your body and mind. Everything starts inside, and that's why you're going to test yourself to see what has gone so wrong in your body. That gives you the leverage to use cellular methods of removing the harmful substances from the very source of your diseases.

Today is the day you throw the foods away that put your body in the shape it is now. You know what you want to achieve. You know what needs to go. Let go of all the products, food and otherwise, that only set your health back and make you grow old before your time. Indeed, you can halt the aging process from inside by adding clean nutrition to your life.

You can remove the symptoms that plagued you with simple methods and mouth-watering recipes straight from my kitchen. The superfoods won't only help to cleanse your body, but they'll also restore valuable nutrients you've lost. Your body and every cell inside of it, ranging from the brain to the feet, will thank you over and over.

Planning your meals has never been easier, and you can apply the natural fasting process to stimulate self-healing and regeneration inside your body. Let's not forget the exercises I've collected for you. You can choose to build muscle, lose weight, or keep your organs as strong as an ox. Everything you've learned goes beyond practical. It also includes enjoyable nutrition, exercises, and mindful practices.

Re-activate your body and mind to heal from the inside out because that's what it was built to do. My experience with my daughter, other kids, and wife has taught me that there's nothing more valuable than health and happiness. The healthier you become, the happier you'll be. I'm rooting for you to achieve the ultimate health my family did.

Now, go out there and make the changes, one step at a time.

Plea From Author

Hey Reader, you got to the end of my book. I hope this means you enjoyed it. Whether or not you did, I would like to thank you for giving me your valuable time to try to entertain you and you found valuable content that was helpful. I'm truly blessed I can have this opportunity, but I only have this opportunity because of people like you; people kind enough to give my books a chance and spend their hard-earned money buying them. For that I'm entirely grateful.

If you would like to find out more about my other books then please visit my website for full details. You can find it at:

www.amazingjaqproducts.com/publishing

Also feel free to come and join our Facebook Group as I would love to have you be part of our growing community that is eager to stay healthy.

www.facebook.com/groups/puresmartlife

If you enjoyed this book and would like to help, then you could think about leaving a review on Amazon or anywhere else that readers visit.

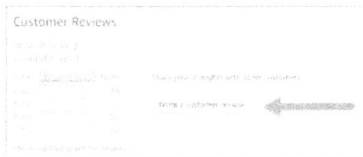

I have posted below the link directly to Amazon as it is always a challenge how to find it on Amazon. The most important part of how a book sells is by how many positive reviews it has, so leave one and you are directly helping me to continue my journey as a full-time author and publisher. Thanks in advance to anyone who does. It means alot!

https://www.amazingjaqproducts.com/review-create/review=1

REFERENCES

Anderson, J., & Burakoff, R. (2020, September 24). *Is GMO wheat increasing celiac disease and gluten sensitivity?* Verywell Health. https://www.verywellhealth.com/is-gmo-wheat-causing-increases-in-gluten-issues-562530

Anthony, K. (2017, December 14). *Heavy metal detox diet.* Healthline. https://www.healthline.com/health/heavy-metal-detox

Back to Health. (n.d.-a). *Testing.* Back to Health Natural Solutions. https://www.backtohealthnaturalsolutions.com/testing/

Back to Health. (2020, November 28). *Eat the right carbs and sleep better.* Back to Health Natural Solutions. https://www.backtohealthnaturalsolutions.com/eat-the-right-carbs-and-sleep-better/

Back To Health Chiropractic Center. (2020). *Chiropractic fights a virus... how?* YouTube. https://www.youtube.com/watch?v=RcfU3rkDn8o

Balfour, L. (2014, August 7). *11 signs it's time to clean up the

toxins in your body. Lifehack. https://www.lifehack.org/
articles/lifestyle/11-signs-its-time-clean-the-toxins-your-
body.html

Bjarnadottir, A., & Seitz, A. (2020, May 14). *Gluten: What is
it and why is it bad for some people?* Medical News Today.
https://www.medicalnewstoday.com/articles/318606

Brown, E. (2016). *What does it mean to eat clean?* Mayo
Clinic.   https://www.mayoclinic.org/healthy-lifestyle/
nutrition-and-healthy-eating/in-depth/what-does-it-mean-
to-eat-clean/art-20270125

Bull, M. J., & Plummer, N. T. (2014). Part I: The human gut
microbiome in health and disease. *Integrative Medicine
(Encinitas, Calif.)*, 13(6), 17–22. https://www.ncbi.nlm.nih.gov/
pmc/articles/PMC4566439

Carpenter, H. (2019, February 28). *14 types of push-ups—
and how they help you.* Outside Online. https://www.
outsideonline.com/2390287/types-of-pushups

Clean & Delicious. (2017). *A beginners guide to healthy
eating | how to eat healthy | 15 tips.* YouTube. https://www.
youtube.com/watch?v=jwWpTAXu-Sg

Cresci, G. A. M., & Izzo, K. (2019). *Gut microbiome - an
overview.* Science Direct. https://www.sciencedirect.com/
topics/medicine-and-dentistry/gut-microbiome#:~:text=
The%20gut%20microbiome%2C%20as%20defined

Defagó, M. D., Elorriaga, N., Irazola, V. E., & Rubinstein,
A. L. (2014). Influence of food patterns on endothelial
biomarkers: A systematic review. *The Journal of Clinical
Hypertension*, 16(12), 907–913. https://doi.org/10.1111/jch.12431

DeLauer, T. (2018). *How to do intermittent fasting: Complete
guide.*   YouTube.   https://www.youtube.com/watch?
v=LLVf3dorqqY

Diet Doctor. (n.d.-b). *500+ easy keto recipes – meals, bread & more.* Diet Doctor. https://www.dietdoctor.com/low-carb/keto/recipes

Dog, T. L. (2014, April 8). *25 healing herbs you can use every day.* Prevention. https://www.prevention.com/life/a20438272/25-healing-herbs-you-can-use-every-day/

Edinburgh, R. M., Hengist, A., Smith, H. A., Travers, R. L., Koumanov, F., Betts, J. A., Thompson, D., Walhin, J.-P., Wallis, G. A., Hamilton, D. L., Stevenson, E. J., Tipton, K. D., & Gonzalez, J. T. (2018). Preexercise breakfast ingestion versus extended overnight fasting increases postprandial glucose flux after exercise in healthy men. *American Journal of Physiology-Endocrinology and Metabolism*, 315(5), E1062–E1074. https://doi.org/10.1152/ajpendo.00163.2018

Editors of Women's Health. (2019a, July 31). *This workout is A serious squat test but your butt will thank you.* Women's Health. https://www.womenshealthmag.com/fitness/a19904135/types-of-squats/

Farkas, D. J. (2019, October 11). *How to stop having pain all over.* Back to Health Natural Solutions. https://www.backtohealthnaturalsolutions.com/how-to-stop-having-pain-all-over/

Farvid, M. S., Chen, W. Y., Michels, K. B., Cho, E., Willett, W. C., & Eliassen, A. H. (2016). Fruit and vegetable consumption in adolescence and early adulthood and risk of breast cancer: Population based cohort study. *BMJ*, i2343. https://doi.org/10.1136/bmj.i2343

Frey, M., & Stanten, M. (2020, October 12). *4 reasons why walking is real exercise.* Verywell Fit. https://www.verywellfit.com/is-walking-a-real-exercise-4058698

Ghaisas, S., Maher, J., & Kanthasamy, A. (2016). Gut

microbiome in health and disease: Linking the microbiome–gut–brain axis and environmental factors in the pathogenesis of systemic and neurodegenerative diseases. *Pharmacology & Therapeutics*, 158, 52–62. https://doi.org/10.1016/j.pharmthera.2015.11.012

Gonzales, X. (2019, November 17). *Low carb vegetables list for keto diet.* All Natural Ideas. https://allnaturalideas.com/low-carb-vegetables-for-keto-diet/#:~:text=Low%20Carb%20Vegetables%20List%20for%20Keto%20Diet.%20The

Gordon, B. (2019, August 20). *Are food sensitivity tests accurate?* Eat Right. https://www.eatright.org/health/allergies-and-intolerances/food-intolerances-and-sensitivities/are-food-sensitivity-tests-accurate#:~:text=In%20the%20case%20of%20food

Hausauer, N. (n.d.). *Basic energy healing techniques.* The Energy Healing Site. https://www.the-energy-healing-site.com/energy-healing-techniques.html

Hills, J. (2014, June 1). *Warning signs your body is overloaded with toxins & how to fix it FAST.* Healthy and Natural World. https://www.healthyandnaturalworld.com/top-signs-your-body-is-toxic-and-what-to-do-about-it/

Julson, E. (2018, July 17). *Master cleanse (lemonade) diet: Does it work for weight loss?* Healthline. https://www.healthline.com/nutrition/master-cleanse-lemonade-diet#how-it-works

Kessler, G. (2016, November 17). *Are there really 10,000 diseases and just 500 'cures'?* The Washington Post. https://www.washingtonpost.com/news/fact-checker/wp/2016/11/17/are-there-really-10000-diseases-and-500-cures/

Live Science Staff. (2006, May 30). *Top 10 Mysterious Diseases.* Live Science. https://www.livescience.com/11333-top-10-mysterious-diseases.html

Livermore, S. (2020, October 5). *35+ keto-friendly breakfasts that'll keep you full all day*. Delish. https://www.delish.com/cooking/g4806/keto-breakfast/

Living Young. (2019b). *Pesticides and processed foods rob the body of nutrients*. Living Young. https://livingyoungcenter.com/pesticides-and-processed-foods-rob-the-body-of-nutrients/

Medicine Plus. (n.d.-c). *What is genetic testing?* Medicine Plus. https://medlineplus.gov/genetics/understanding/testing/genetictesting/

Mindvalley. (2019, May 16). *The complete guide to the 7 chakras - for beginners*. Mindvalley Blog. https://blog.mindvalley.com/7-chakras/

Mindworks Team. (2018, July 11). *What is zen meditation? Benefits & techniques*. Mindworks Meditation. https://mindworks.org/blog/what-is-zen-meditation-benefits-techniques/

Minnis, G., & Conkleton, E. (2020, January 21). *Cycling benefits: 11 reasons cycling is good for you*. Healthline. https://www.healthline.com/health/fitness-exercise/cycling-benefits

Moro, T., Tinsley, G., Bianco, A., Marcolin, G., Pacelli, Q. F., Battaglia, G., Palma, A., Gentil, P., Neri, M., & Paoli, A. (2016). Effects of eight weeks of time-restricted feeding (16/8) on basal metabolism, maximal strength, body composition, inflammation, and cardiovascular risk factors in resistance-trained males. *Journal of Translational Medicine*, 14(1). https://doi.org/10.1186/s12967-016-1044-0

National Health Council. (2014). *About chronic diseases*. https://doi.org/10.1056/NEJMsa022615

O'Neill, M. (2020, May 21). *Some children are developing a mysterious new illness that could be caused by COVID-19.*

Health. https://www.health.com/condition/infectious-diseases/coronavirus/mysterious-illness-children-covid-19

Philp, T. (2019, July 18). *Adrenal fatigue and stress testing - complete guide (2019)*. Healthpath. https://healthpath.com/adrenal/adrenal-fatigue-test-guide-2019/

Pietrocola, F., Malik, S. A., Mariño, G., Vacchelli, E., Senovilla, L., chaba, kariman, Niso-Santano, M., Maiuri, M. C., Madeo, F., & Kroemer, G. (2014). Coffee induces autophagy in vivo. *Cell Cycle*, 13(12), 1987–1994. https://doi.org/10.4161/cc.28929

Pompa, D. (2015, July 23). *True cellular detox - top 5 strategies to create your best health ever*. Dr. Pompa & Cellular Healing TV. https://drpompa.com/cellular-detox/true-cellular-detox-a-top-5-strategy-to-create-your-best-health-ever/

Rooted in Rest. (2016). *How I meal plan and shop once every two weeks (whole and organic on a budget)*. YouTube. https://www.youtube.com/watch?v=I0A4xCKFwgA

Samuel, E., C.S.C.S., Williams, B., & NASM. (2020, April 12). *55 resistance band moves you can do at home*. Men's Health. https://www.menshealth.com/fitness/a32093962/resistance-band-workouts/

Sass, C. (2013, July 18). *Planning a detox or juice cleanse? 5 dos and don'ts*. Health. https://www.health.com/nutrition/planning-a-detox-or-juice-cleanse-5-dos-and-donts

Splitzler, F. (2019, April 8). *11 simple ways to start clean eating today*. Healthline. https://www.healthline.com/nutrition/11-ways-to-eat-clean#:~:text=%2011%20Simple%20Ways%20to%20Start%20Clean%20Eating

Vertex Software Corporation. (n.d.-d). *Neurotransmitter testing*. Neurogistics. https://www.neurogistics.com/products/

neurotransmitter-testing#:~:text=A%20neurotransmitter%
20test%20provides%20information

Vibrant Wellness. (n.d.-e). *Environmental toxins*. Vibrant Wellness. https://www.vibrant-wellness.com/tests/
environmental-toxins/#:~:text=Environmental%
20ToxinsTo%20test%20for

Wikipedia Contributors. (2019, April 11). *Zen*. Wikipedia. https://en.wikipedia.org/wiki/Zen

Wong, C. (2004, June 3). *Complementary and alternative medicine use in the U.S.* Verywell Health. https://www.verywellhealth.com/alternative-medicine-usage-in-the-us-88732

Wood, J. (2019). *What to eat for a flat stomach | vegan meal plan*. YouTube. https://www.youtube.com/watch?v=b5E3yGsjat4

Yuen, C., & Bubnis, D. (2018, July 20). *Foam rolling: 8 magic moves that'll relax all the tension in your*. Healthline. https://www.healthline.com/health/fitness-exercise/foam-rolling-how-to

Zyrowski, N. (n.d.). *True cellular detox: 90 day detox kit*. NuVision Health Center. https://store.nuvisionhealthcenter.com/products/true-cellular-detox-90-day-detox-kit

Image References

Chakra Stream. (n.d.). Pixabay. https://pixabay.com/photos/
spiritualism-awakening-meditation-4552237/

Chiropractor. (n.d.) Unsplash. https://unsplash.com/
photos/hBLf2nvp-Yc

Gut Bacteria. (n.d). Pixabay. https://pixabay.com/photos/
bacteria-medical-biology-health-3658992/

Herbs. (n.d.). Unsplash. https://unsplash.com/photos/d5xQVtmTUeo

Pesticides. (n.d.). Pixabay. https://pixabay.com/photos/farmer-tractor-agriculture-farm-880567/

Quinoa Salad Variation. (n.d.). Pixabay. https://pixabay.com/photos/pan-quinoa-colorful-vegetables-1832926/

Resistance Bands. (n.d.). Unsplash. https://unsplash.com/photos/rWBBDErPXcY

www.ingramcontent.com/pod-product-compliance
Lightning Source LLC
Chambersburg PA
CBHW020257030426
42336CB00010B/803